Praise for *Yoga for Fibromyalgia*

Shoosh Lettick Crotzer has written a wonderful guide for women with fibromyalgia. It is not only clear that she understands the health issues of patients, but also clear that she understands the benefits of empowering women to take charge of their health. I love the emphasis on how to apply principles of yoga to everyday life. This book is packed with practical advice and I will recommend it to my patients.

—Leslie J. Crofford, M.D., Univeristy of Kentucky; Gloria W. Singletary Professor; Chief, Division of Rheumatology and Women's Health; Director, Center for the Advancement of Women's Health

Shoosh is a healer. She shares techniques and gifted insights honed and focused for a lifetime. In *Yoga for Fibromyalgia,* she gives practical ways to relieve pain, improve mobility, and restore health. Share it with a loved one in need.

—Ganga White, author of *Yoga Beyond Belief: Insights to Awaken and Deepen Your Practice*

This book offers clear and relevant yoga and lifestyle information to those suffering from fibromyalgia. But it offers something even more important: hope that things can get better. Highly recommended for yoga teachers, for experienced yoga students, and for those people just beginning to practice.

—Judith Hanson Lasater, Ph.D., P.T., author of *30 Essential Yoga Poses: For Beginning Students and Their Teachers*

Shoosh Lettick Crotzer understands that most people with fibromyalgia can benefit from a gentle approach to yoga. In this book, she teaches a variety of helpful poses and visualization techniques; suggests practice routines to meet your changing needs; and, most important for healing, guides you toward making yoga part of your everyday life.

—Timothy McCall, M.D., medical editor of *Yoga Journal*; author of *Yoga as Medicine: The Yogic Prescription for Health and Healing*

This book is an inviting introduction to yoga for fibromyalgia sufferers. With a well-considered series of gentle stretches and breathing and relaxation exercises, this program is beneficial even for more debilitated beginners and forms a foundation for those students ready to move on to other active yoga poses.

—Julie Gudmestad, P.T., director, Gudmestad Yoga Studio, Portland, Oregon; author of *Yoga Journal*'s "Anatomy" column

Ms. Crotzer's breathing and awareness techniques are excellent for increasing focus and mental clarity, which facilitate coping not only with fibromyalgia but also with general stress. She has done a terrific job of adapting traditional yoga poses, some of which can be done in a chair. And the book's instructions and photos make the poses easy to follow. I particularly like the sections called "Everyday Yoga" (at the end of each pose), which give examples of how to use the poses throughout the day. Her yoga sequences can clearly help people with fibromyalgia in a way that is gentle and does not cause pain.

—Jeanne Melvin, M.S., OTR/L, FAOTA, author of *Fibromyalgia Syndrome, Getting Healthy*; in practice at Solutions for Wellness, Santa Monica, CA

Yoga for Fibromyalgia

Rodmell Press Yoga Shorts

By Sandy Blaine
Yoga for Computer Users
Yoga for Healthy Knees

By Shoosh Lettick Crotzer
Yoga for Fibromyalgia

By Judith Hanson Lasater, Ph.D., P.T.
Yoga Abs
Yoga for Pregnancy

rodmell press

YOGA SHORTS

YOGA

FOR FIBROMYALGIA

MOVE, BREATHE, AND RELAX
TO IMPROVE YOUR QUALITY OF LIFE

▼   ▼   ▼   ▼   ▼   ▼   ▼   ▼   ▼   ▼

Shoosh Lettick Crotzer

RODMELL PRESS   BERKELEY, CALIFORNIA, 2008

Library of Congress Cataloging-in-Publication Data

Crotzer, Shoosh Lettick, 1950-
  Yoga for fibromyalgia : move, breathe, and relax to improve your quality of life /
Shoosh Lettick Crotzer. -- 1st ed.
      p. cm. — (Rodmell Press yoga shorts)
  Includes bibliographical references and index.
  ISBN-13: 978-1-930485-16-7 (pbk. : alk. paper)
  ISBN-10: 1-930485-16-6 (pbk. : alk. paper)
  1. Fibromyalgia—Alternative treatment. 2. Yoga—Therapeutic use. I. Title.
  RC927.3.C76 2008
  616.7'420642—dc22
                            2007047904

Printed and bound in China
First edition

ISBN-10: 1-930485-16-6
ISBN-13: 978-1-930485-16-7

10 09 08 1 2 3 4 5 6 7 8 9 10

Editor: Linda Cogozzo   Photographs: David Martinez, Inc.
Associate Editor: Holly Hammond   Lithographer: Kwong Fat Offset Printing Co., Ltd.
Indexer: Ty Koontz   Text set in Dante
Design: Gopa & Ted2, Inc.   Distributed by Publishers Group West

For Bonnie, who has spent many years coping with fibromyalgia. I hope this book helps provide some relief for you and many others.

Contents

▼ ▼ ▼ ▼ ▼ ▼ ▼

Acknowledgments

▼ ▼ ▼ ▼ ▼ ▼ ▼ ▼ ▼ ▼ ▼

I began practicing yoga in 1974 with my first teacher, Sambhu, and I maintain a thankful place in my heart for his gift to me. Through him I met Ganga White, who has become a friend as well as a teacher. I take students to his White Lotus Foundation annually for a private class and discussion with him and his wonderful partner and wife, Tracey Rich. They remain models for me of blending the practice of yoga with the art of living yoga.

In 1976 I studied in Ann Arbor, Michigan, with some of B. K. S. Iyengar's devoted students, who were responsible for bringing him and his yoga to the United States. From them, I learned the foundation of my own yoga. Mr. Iyengar's contributions to yoga are invaluable.

One of my most influential teachers does not teach yoga. I call Dr. John Hannon the "Zen master of body workers." He taught me new ways to understand my own body and then guided me to keep making new discoveries. This changed my yoga practice and the way I teach yoga in an unexpected and exciting manner. Not a day goes by that I don't thank him. John also gave me valuable pointers in reviewing the early drafts of this book, for which I am grateful.

Donna Everix also reviewed this book. Her knowledge as a physical therapist specializing in arthritis and fibromyalgia has been a guiding light for me since we worked together on *Yoga for Arthritis*. She was the Arthritis Foundation's consultant on that project, and we have been friends and colleagues since.

Dr. Barry Dorfman, a psychiatrist, along with his wife, Leabah Winter, who has fibromyalgia, also were instrumental in helping me fine-tune this book. We spent many hours discussing and rewriting, and I am sincerely indebted to them for their help.

Joni Hunt, yoga student, editor, and friend, graciously helped me with her editing skills. I owe her many thanks.

My brother David Lettick, an artist and writer, reviewed the first draft in great detail, offering me insights and useful edits. I am lucky to have a close-knit and supportive family, including my husband, Colby. I thank them for their advice, encouragement, and love.

I thank Donald Moyer and Linda Cogozzo at Rodmell Press for inspiring me to write this book. Their educated and patient assistance helped create this final edition.

Most important of all, I thank my students for teaching me what they need.

Foreword

▼ ▼ ▼ ▼ ▼ ▼ ▼ ▼ ▼ ▼

In *Yoga for Fibromyalgia*, Shoosh Lettick Crotzer has skillfully adapted the traditional practice of yoga asana (poses) to the needs of those with the painful, chronic condition of fibromyalgia. It is a condition I know well, and I was pleased to serve as the model for the poses in the book.

When I experienced my first symptoms of fibromyalgia, about eighteen years ago, I was a yoga teacher and a professional dancer. Even though I had been giving private yoga sessions to students with chronic fatigue syndrome, which some consider to be related to or the same as fibromyalgia, I did not at that time recognize what the sudden onset of fatigue, pain, dizziness, and a host of other symptoms meant for me. Nor did my doctor.

Over the next fifteen years, the symptoms came and went, triggered by encounters with various stressors. I learned that this particular constellation of symptoms was indicative of fibromyalgia, and that there was, at that time, no definitive treatment for it. I continued to practice and teach yoga in accord with my pain and energy levels. When I was ill, my practice emphasized rest in supported and basic supine postures, which gently eased the painfully tight muscles, decreased inflammation, and restored deep sleep. When I was well, a more active practice rebalanced and strengthened the affected muscle groups and realigned my posture. I lived an almost "normal" life.

I believe Shoosh's presentation of yoga poses, specifically adapted for fibromyalgia, can help those who also have this painful condition find ease, balance, rest, and hope. I encourage those who teach yoga to people with fibromyalgia to study and consider incorporating Shoosh's approach into their teaching practice, and I strongly recommend *Yoga for Fibromyalgia* as a resource for all who care for those with fibromyalgia—family members, friends, caregivers, doctors, and physical therapists.

May all those living with fibromyalgia experience ease, vitality, and the fullness of life!

Deirdre Carrigan

Green Gulch Farm, Muir Beach, CA

October 31, 2007

Part I:

Fibromyalgia and Yoga

▼   ▼   ▼   ▼   ▼   ▼   ▼   ▼   ▼   ▼   ▼

I STARTED PRACTICING YOGA when I was in my early twenties. I loved the challenge, strength, and beauty of the poses and the techniques that showed me how to breathe properly and relax. Since I was also a special education teacher at the time, I naturally began to teach some of these skills to my students. My background teaching yoga to both children and adults with various disabilities has now expanded to include those with multiple sclerosis, arthritis, and cancer. In 1997 I created a program and video for the Arthritis Foundation that included specific pointers for those with fibromyalgia. I have continued working with students and their fibromyalgia symptoms to develop the adaptive yoga poses included in this book. Just as they continue to help my students, I hope they provide you with relief in coping with the physical, mental, and emotional challenges of fibromyalgia

What Is Fibromyalgia?

Fibromyalgia is an arthritis-related condition characterized by chronic muscular pain and stiffness, aches, soft tissue tenderness, headaches, dizziness, nausea, cognitive impairment, general fatigue, disturbed sleep, and more. Its causes are unknown, so it is referred to as a syndrome rather than a disease. It affects approximately 11 million people in the United States, 900,000 in Canada, and 6 million in Europe. They are mostly women between the ages of thirty and fifty. Tests can rule out other disorders, but there is no one specific test that can confirm fibromyalgia. In 1990 the American College of Rheumatology, the organization of doctors who treat arthritis and related conditions, presented criteria for diagnosing it. The criteria include having pain in eleven out of eighteen tender-point sites, along with general chronic pain for at least three months. (See Figure A and Figure B.)

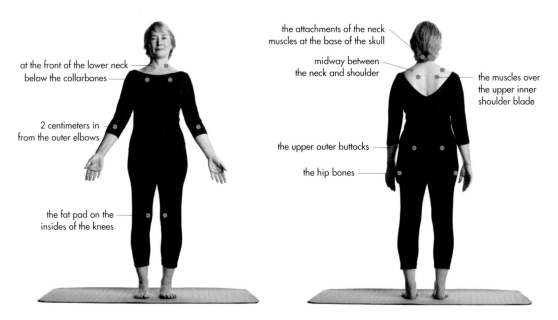

the attachments of the neck muscles at the base of the skull

midway between the neck and shoulder

the muscles over the upper inner shoulder blade

at the front of the lower neck below the collarbones

2 centimeters in from the outer elbows

the upper outer buttocks

the hip bones

the fat pad on the insides of the knees

FIGURE A TENDER-POINT SITES, FRONT VIEW

FIGURE B TENDER-POINT SITES, BACK VIEW

Yoga and Fibromyalgia

Yoga is an art and science that began in the Indus Valley civilization thousands of years ago and is now firmly rooted in the West. The word *yoga* comes from Sanskrit, an ancient Indian language, and means "union": of the body, the mind, and the spirit. The most common Western interpretation focuses on refining the body, mind, and spirit through poses, called *asana,* combined with breathing techniques, called *pranamaya.*

Yoga's physical practices are noncompetitive and adaptable to any individual, including those with special needs, such as fibromyalgia. They provide another potential treatment option for those with physical difficulties. Alignment is emphasized, so posture and balance may improve. Yoga teaches the practitioner where muscles are located and how to strengthen and stretch them. You can learn how to release tension, allowing the body to feel more energized. Yoga also includes relaxation techniques that can reduce stress.

In *Exercise and Fibromyalgia,* Mark J. Pellegrino, M.D., says, "Because fibromyalgia muscles are so tight, they are more vulnerable to sprains and strains, so it is especially important that this tightness be counteracted by stretching." Yoga can teach you how to stretch to relieve tension and stiffness in specific muscles. With yoga movement and breathing, visualization, and relaxation techniques, pain and fatigue can be reduced, deeper sleep can be achieved, and stress can be eased. Inappropriate exercises can result in increased distress, but there should be no adverse side effects from adapted yoga. Most people feel better right away after a yoga session. My students often report that they are sleeping better, they have less tension in their muscles, and they have learned ways to cope with stress. They tell me that yoga has improved their quality of life.

General Guidelines

I know you are eager to get started, but resist jumping ahead to the sequences in part 3, and take the time to peruse the entire book first. That way, you can familiarize yourself with the material, which will enhance a safe and satisfying experience of the poses. Here are some points to keep in mind as you practice yoga with this book.

You are responsible for your own body. Not all poses and techniques are appropriate for everyone, so before starting, talk with your doctor or health care provider about which poses and exercises would be best for you and which you should avoid. Then listen to what your body tells you. If a pose or an exercise doesn't feel right, do not do it. But at the same time, don't be afraid of working to make changes. (See part 3, "Practicing Yoga for Fibromyalgia," for more tips on practicing safely.)

Understand the difference between a tight muscle and a tense muscle. When you exercise, you are consciously tightening (contracting) and strengthening specific muscles. Muscles also tighten from inactivity. Sitting all day, for example, tightens the backs of your thighs. To relieve a tight muscle, you stretch it. On the other hand, tense muscles come from unconscious movement. When you are driving your car, for example, and your shoulders rise toward your ears in a traffic jam, you are not intentionally doing neck-strengthening exercises. To relieve a tense muscle, you need to relax it first and then stretch it. If you try to stretch a tense muscle, you can damage it, because part of your brain unconsciously tells your muscle to tighten, while the conscious part tells it to stretch, resulting in a tug-of-war effect.

To avoid this conflict, it is vital to recognize the difference between tense and tight and to learn how to relax before stretching. The act of releasing a tense muscle in itself is not difficult. You just let go. But what is not so easy is learning where the muscle tension is and isolating it so it can be relaxed. With time and awareness, this becomes easier.

Begin and end with the foundation. Each pose or exercise has a foundation, which varies from pose to pose, exercise to exercise. In standing poses, your foundation is your feet. Make sure you are standing correctly, with your feet lined up, not turned out or staggered, one more forward than the other. You then work up from your feet to align the rest of your body.

In sitting poses, your hips and pelvis are the foundation, so make sure you start your pose balanced evenly on each side of your buttocks, with both hips level and aligned. If your foundation is out of alignment when you begin a pose, it can nullify any benefits the pose might have offered and possibly provoke other problems.

When you complete a pose or exercise, remember to focus on your foundation once again, to make sure you end up in alignment.

How to Use This Book

This book is not intended to be a diagnostic tool, nor does it offer any cures. However, I want to help you find ways to improve your quality of life by reducing stress, pain, fatigue, and muscle stiffness and by getting deeper sleep. I specifically chose the yoga poses for this book as the most appropriate ones for you to learn. They do not represent the complete range of possible poses for those with fibromyalgia.

I encourage yoga teachers, doctors, physical therapists, and other health care providers to use this book as a guide when working with their students and patients. If you are reading this book because a loved one has fibromyalgia, then I hope you find these gentle practices and lifestyle tips helpful in extending your care and support. And for all of you lending a hand, you can do the poses too, especially Relaxation Pose (Figure 24)!

The book is organized into four parts. Part 1 includes information on fibromyalgia, yoga, and general guidelines. Part 2, "Yoga Poses for Fibromyalgia," explains how to do the poses, which include standing, seated, and reclining poses, stretches for the upper and lower body, and guided relaxation. Deirdre Carrigan models the poses in the photographs. She has fibromyalgia and is also a yoga teacher who knows firsthand the benefits yoga can provide.

In part 3, "Practicing Yoga for Fibromyalgia," I give guidelines to get you started, such as where and when to practice, what to wear, and the props you will need, as well as sequences for general pain relief and for reducing fatigue and improving sleep, a visualization for pain relief, and routines for maintenance. Part 4, "Living with Fibromyalgia," discusses the importance of deep sleep and ways to improve it, healthy nutrition basics, appropriate physical activities and daily life movement, and psychological well-being.

Use this book in the ways that best serve your day-to-day needs. Appreciate your progress, and enjoy the relief you feel. And don't forget to smile! It's always healing.

Part II:

Yoga Poses for Fibromyalgia

▼　▼　▼　▼　▼　▼　▼　▼　▼　▼

THIS SECTION DESCRIBES how to practice poses and breathing techniques that I recommend for those with fibromyalgia. Some asanas have variations, including those practiced seated. These might be more appropriate for you, so make sure you look through the entire section before beginning your practice. In part 3, you'll find important guidelines to help your practice. Make sure you read them before you begin the poses. Part 3 also includes sequences to relieve pain, improve sleep and reduce fatigue, and maintain flexibility and body awareness.

Above the name of each pose, I have noted whether it is an asana, an exercise, or pranayama. The asana names are given in English and also in Sanskrit. The overall benefits of the asanas are followed by the foundation of each pose, cautions (when required), and lists of props you will need and some you might need. Guided instructions come next. At the end of each pose, a section called "Everyday Yoga" gives you some ideas for integrating the pose into your ordinary activities.

Let the poses teach you how to feel better. We begin with a position to teach you how to sit properly and follow that with a breathing routine. These will be useful for many other poses in this book. Remember to enjoy your practice and respect the limits your body may require.

Seated Mountain Pose

▼ ▼ ▼ ▼ ▼ ▼ ▼ ALIGNS THE SPINE • RELEASES LOWER
ABDOMINAL TENSION • RELIEVES LOWER BACK PAIN

FOUNDATION: Pelvis

PROPS: 1 nonskid mat • 1 chair

POSSIBLE PROP: 1 blanket or pillow

The spinal column is composed of twenty-four vertebrae that form three grace-ful curves: at the lower back, at the middle back, and at the neck. To stand or sit well, it is essential to maintain these curves. Why? Alignment, or good pos-ture, is key in maintaining your health. As a result of bad habits and the weight of everyday life, many of us suffer the effects of bad posture, such as shallow breathing, compressed organs, and muscular tension. And if you have fibro-myalgia, optimal postural alignment is even more important to help prevent symptomatic muscle pain.

We will work on improving your posture with Seated Mountain Pose (Fig-ure 1). When standing or seated, your hips and pelvis are the spine's founda-tion. We'll start by aligning them. Place your chair at the edge of your mat. Sit toward the front edge of the chair seat, with your spine lengthened and your knees and feet about hip-width apart. Place your feet on the mat, directly below

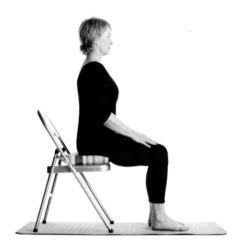

FIGURE 1
SEATED MOUNTAIN POSE

your knees, not angled out or in or one forward of the other.

Your abdomen can relax more if your knees are angled slightly below your hips. If they are not, sit higher by putting a folded blanket or pillow on the chair seat. Rest your hands on your thighs, palms down, relaxed.

Relax and release your shoulders down, away from your ears. Let your elbows feel heavy, and soften your abdomen. Bring your awareness to your sitting bones, which are the two bony structures at the base of your pelvis that you are sitting on. It is common to tilt the top of the pelvis back and roll onto the buttocks. This forces the lower back, which normally curves inward, to curve outward. When this happens, it feels as if there is a thread running from your navel through your torso that is being pulled from behind your back. Sitting this way is a common cause of lower back pain, so we'll work to correct this misalignment.

You can learn what it feels like to be in alignment by consciously being out of it. Roll back onto your buttocks, and notice what happens to your posture. You slouch, your shoulders round forward, your chest contracts, your chin moves forward, and you compress the back of your neck. Now roll forward onto the center of your sitting bones. Feel how the spine lengthens and seems lighter. Your chest opens, your chin moves back, and the back of your neck lengthens.

Do it again. Sitting in alignment takes less effort and reduces muscle tension in the hips and pelvis. You may experience a feeling of melting release in your abdomen. It can also make your back feel less tired.

With attention and practice, you will learn to feel when you are properly aligned. Are you leaning forward? Is there more weight on one sitting bone than the other? Are you slouching? Gently adjust your position to reestablish your natural spinal curves.

Now bring your awareness to your neck and your head. Quietly move your chin forward, then draw it back, lengthening the front and back of your neck evenly. Come to the spot where your head feels balanced on your neck, and let it rest there. Relax the muscles in your face and release your jaw, separating your upper and lower teeth.

We will practice Seated Mountain Pose as the foundation of many of the poses and exercises in this book, such as Seated Eagle Pose (Figure 7A and Figure 7B) and Seated Twist Pose (Figure 18A and Figure 18B).

Everyday Yoga

You can practice Seated Mountain Pose during your daily activities or any time you are seated. For example, when at a computer, start with Seated Mountain Pose. You will be pleasantly surprised at how much longer you can sit without getting tired. Also, when sitting at the dinner table, Seated Mountain Pose can improve your digestion by making sure your organs are not compressed.

Breathing Awareness
SAMA VRTTI

▼ ▼ ▼ ▼ ▼ ▼ ▼ LOWERS BLOOD PRESSURE
• IMPROVES CIRCULATION • REDUCES STRESS • MANAGES PAIN

FOUNDATION: Pelvis

PRACTICE WITH CARE: If you feel breathless, anxious, light-headed,
or nauseous during Breathing Awareness, let your breath return to normal.
Rest for several cycles of breath before resuming Breathing Awareness
or just stop. You can try it again on another day.

PROPS: 1 nonskid mat • 1 chair

POSSIBLE PROP: 1 blanket or pillow

The breath: so simple, so accessible! Yet many of us primarily use the top one-third of our lungs when we breathe. Physically, when you inhale, your abdomen and chest expand, and when you exhale, they contract. By learning to draw the breath into the middle and bottom of the lungs, you can increase your lung capacity simply by using more of them. This is positive for those with fibromyalgia because it can reduce stress and help you cope with pain.

Just as asanas teach us to move consciously, pranayama guides us to breathe with awareness. When you open your chest or arch your back in a pose, you will inhale. When you compress or close your chest, such as in forward bending movements, you will exhale. Eventually this will come naturally with your movements. To begin to develop this breathing, I have found it beneficial to start my students with a gentle but deep practice called Breathing Awareness. You can practice it in several ways.

In Seated Mountain Pose. Set up in Seated Mountain Pose (Figure 1), sitting on a folded blanket or a pillow, if you need one. Take your time to settle yourself and establish your alignment. Place one hand lightly on your abdomen, below your ribs but above your navel, and the other hand on your thigh, palm down, relaxed (Figure 2A). Soften your face, your jaw, your throat. Allow your gaze to be soft.

Unless you are congested, always breathe through your nose. Inhale slowly and gently, and feel your hand move out as your abdomen expands. Then, as you exhale slowly, feel your hand move toward your spine. This is deep

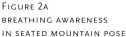
FIGURE 2A
BREATHING AWARENESS
IN SEATED MOUNTAIN POSE

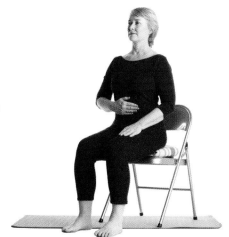

abdominal breathing. The lungs have more capillaries at their base, so taking deeper breaths, drawing more air toward the bottom of your lungs, is a more efficient way for you to get oxygen into your bloodstream. This is beneficial for those with fibromyalgia because it can help reduce fatigue and promote deeper sleep.

Repeat for 10 breaths. If this feels like a strain, then repeat for as many times as you can without force. Your capacity will increase with practice.

In Relaxation Pose. If you find it uncomfortable to practice Breathing Awareness in Seated Mountain Pose, you can lie in Relaxation Pose (Figure 24), either on the floor or in bed or on a sofa. When you place your hand on your abdomen, your hand will rise and fall when you breathe, instead of moving in and out (Figure 2B). You can use the counting or visualization techniques that follow to help you relax or fall asleep. As you will discover, this is a simple but very rewarding practice.

FIGURE 2B
BREATHING AWARENESS IN RELAXATION POSE

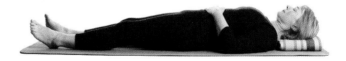

Counting. One way to practice Breathing Awareness is to inhale and exhale while counting silently. This can be done either in Seated Mountain Pose or

Relaxation Pose. Start inhaling to a slow count of 5, and then exhale to a similar count of 5. (If 5 is too much, start with a lesser count.) After repeating the 5 count 3 times, allow your breathing to return to normal for several rounds. Return to the 5 count when you feel ready. Continue to alternate rounds of counting with rounds of normal breathing.

Over the coming days or weeks, increase the count to 6, and repeat 3 times, alternating counting with normal breathing. Once the 6 count is established, you can increase it to 7. Continue to increase the count as high as you want. *Remember, never force the breath.*

Visualization. To deepen your breathing even further, you can focus on feeling the breath move from the bottom of your lungs, into the middle, and then spread out into the upper chest. Whether you are sitting or lying down, this can feel like a warm liquid moving from the center outward. Make sure you keep your shoulders relaxed, and breathe from within. Be creative with your visualizations. Relax.

Everyday Yoga

Practice Breathing Awareness anywhere, anytime: to relax after a stressful day or to center yourself in a challenging situation, such as during a doctor's appointment. Allow the practice to help you listen to your body.

Mountain Pose

TADASANA

▼ ▼ ▼ ▼ ▼ ▼ IMPROVES POSTURE AND BALANCE
• BRINGS STILLNESS

FOUNDATION: **Feet**

PRACTICE WITH CARE: **If you have low blood pressure,
sit down if you start to feel light-headed.**

PROP: **1 nonskid mat**

POSSIBLE PROPS: **a sofa or a chair**

Mountain Pose (Figure 3A) is practiced
standing. (If you prefer, you can work in
Seated Mountain Pose [Figure 1], following
the guided instructions.) It might be helpful to have someone read the instructions
aloud or to record yourself reading them.
That way, you will be able to focus more
intently on the pose.

When practicing asanas, always begin
by focusing on your foundation. In this
asana, your feet are your base of support,

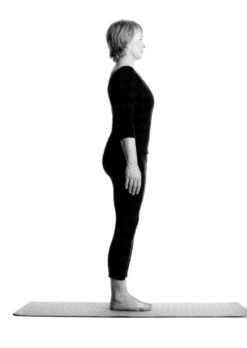

so remove your shoes and socks to let the tactile sensations in your feet assist you. It is best to practice with your mat on a hard floor, because carpet is not stable.

If you feel unsteady, you can stand with your calves against a sofa or with your hands on the back of a chair. Remember, your need for support may change from day to day or within a given day.

Stand on your mat, with your feet a few inches apart and your arms at your sides. If possible, keep your eyes closed. Otherwise, focus on one spot in front of you to keep your eyes still, which will help your balance. Feel the contact of your feet against the mat and the support you receive from the floor. Let your feet feel heavy.

Move your focus up to your legs. Do not lock your knees; feel your legs supported by your feet and ankles. Then move your focus to your pelvis—the area around your abdomen, hips, buttocks, and lower back—and sense the support the pelvis receives from your legs, ankles, and feet. Are your hips balanced? Does one side feel lower than the other? Does one side feel more forward than the other? What can you do to bring yourself into balance?

Let the tension in your buttocks, lower back, and abdomen release. When you do, your navel will feel as if it drops forward and down. This is a subtle movement, which does not come from arching your lower back. Instead, on each exhalation, feel a heaviness and softness in your lower abdomen.

Observe the position of your spine. Does it feel erect and lengthened, or

OPPOSITE:
FIGURE 3A
MOUNTAIN POSE

curved to one side, or slumped forward? What can you do to bring it into balance? How can you use the support of your feet, ankles, legs, and pelvis to do so?

With each exhalation, soften the upper back muscles and relax your shoulders. Do not pull them back, just let them drop, and feel the weight of your arms hanging at your sides. Let your hands feel heavy. With each inhalation, feel your upper body expand and open.

Continue from your spine up into your neck to your head. Move your chin forward gently, and then draw it back, as you lengthen the back of your neck and your throat. Find the spot where your head feels balanced on your neck, and let it rest there. Relax the muscles in your eyes and face and release your jaw, gently separating your upper and lower teeth.

Shift your body weight slightly forward, onto the balls of your feet, without lifting your heels. Then shift your weight back onto your heels, keeping your toes on the floor. Finally, find a spot between your heels and toes where you feel centered.

Focus your attention on your breath. With each inhalation, feel the energy rise evenly on both sides of your spine, toward the top of your head. Lengthen your spine, rising upward like a mountain from its base toward the sky. When you exhale, be aware of your feet in contact with the floor, and let them feel heavy and stable, supported like a mountain by its base. Finally, visualize a thread running from the top of your head, down through your body, to a spot between your feet. See how still you can stand around this thread, without the feeling of swaying. Hold Mountain Pose for 10 gentle breaths. On the 11th breath, inhale your arms out to the sides and straight up, elbows by your ears

(Figure 3B). Keep your shoulders relaxed down from your ears. On the exhalation, gradually lower your arms out to the sides, feeling your hands slowly moving through space until they come to rest at your sides. Stay in this position for one more breath before coming out of the pose. You'll be amazed at how relaxed and strong you will feel.

Everyday Yoga

Remember to practice Mountain Pose when you are especially harried or tense, or when you are standing in a line and feel impatient. It is an easy way to realign and refresh, both physically and mentally.

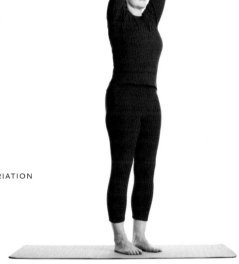

FIGURE 3B
MOUNTAIN POSE, VARIATION

Neck Rotation Stretch

▼   ▼   ▼   ▼   ▼   ▼   INCREASES RANGE OF MOTION IN THE NECK
• RELIEVES NECK TENSION AND PAIN • IMPROVES POSTURE

FOUNDATION: **Pelvis**

PRACTICE WITH CARE: **If you have any diagnosed disk problems
in your neck or feel discomfort in this pose, skip it for now,
and discuss it with your doctor or therapist.**

PROPS: **1 nonskid mat • 1 chair**

POSSIBLE PROP: **1 blanket or pillow**

Many of us unconsciously tense our necks when we're driving or working at
the computer, when we're reading, when we're feeling emotional, and even
when we're trying to stretch or strengthen other parts of our bodies. These
gentle and easy stretches release neck tension and help to maintain full range
of motion. The neck is capable of moving in six directions. It rotates, it moves
forward and back, and it moves side to side. This first simple stretch can gently
help lengthen your neck muscles and reduce neck pain and tension. Two more
neck stretches follow this one.

   Begin in Seated Mountain Pose (Figure 1). Sit on a folded blanket or pillow,
if you need one. As you inhale, turn your head slowly toward the right (Figure
4). Feel your chest expand, drop your shoulders, and keep your chin level. Do

not strain or try to move too far, but rather let your neck lead and the head follow, as opposed to your chin trying to push you farther. On an exhalation, focus on keeping your shoulders relaxed and softening your neck and shoulder muscles. When you inhale, allow your neck to turn; focus on expanding the muscles along the left side of your neck. When you exhale, soften and relax the pose. Hold this pose for 3 breaths, exhale back to the center, and then repeat on the other side. A variation is to hold each side for just 1 breath and repeat the series, side to side, 3 times.

Everyday Yoga

As you might imagine, the uses of Neck Rotation Stretch are many: as a morning stretch, sitting on the side of your bed; at your computer; at a stop light; waiting for an appointment; at the movies. Practicing will increase your comfort when sitting.

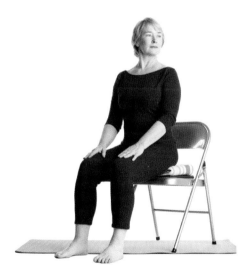

FIGURE 4
NECK ROTATION STRETCH

Forward-and-Back Neck Stretch

▼ ▼ ▼ ▼ ▼ ▼ ▼ INCREASES RANGE OF MOTION IN THE FRONT
AND BACK OF THE NECK • RELIEVES NECK TENSION AND PAIN
• IMPROVES POSTURE

FOUNDATION: **Pelvis**

PRACTICE WITH CARE: **If you have any diagnosed disk problems in your neck
or feel discomfort in this pose, skip it for now, and discuss it with your doctor or
therapist.**

PROPS: **1 nonskid mat • 1 chair**

POSSIBLE PROP: **1 blanket or pillow**

Begin in Seated Mountain Pose (Figure 1). Sit on a folded blanket or pillow, if
you need one. Rest your hands on your thighs, palms down, relaxed. Take the
time that you need to establish this foundation pose. We'll practice Forward-
and-Back Neck Stretch in two stages. In stage 1, you lengthen the muscles in
the back of your neck. In stage 2, the throat area opens.

Stage 1. Inhale and, on the exhalation, slowly lower your chin toward your
chest. Be careful not to collapse the breastbone, ribs, or diaphragm. Relax your
shoulders, and keep your spine lengthened. On an inhalation, stretch both arms
overhead, and interlock your fingers. On the exhalation, lower your hands onto
your head, placing them a bit behind the crown, with your elbows dropping

down toward your thighs (Figure 5A). Feel the weight of your hands and arms. Keep your shoulders relaxed down from your ears, and soften your abdomen. On an inhalation, bring the breath into the back of your neck, and focus on expanding the muscles there. Then exhale and soften those muscles. Hold this pose for 3 breaths. On the last exhalation, lower your arms to their resting position on your thighs. Lift your head. Rest in Seated Mountain Pose.

Stage 2. The most important aspect to this phase is ease. Do not force or strain. To balance the forward movement of stage 1, inhale, lift your chin, and look up (Figure 5B). Don't push your head back; keep your jaw relaxed. Lengthen the front of your neck as you keep your shoulders relaxed down from

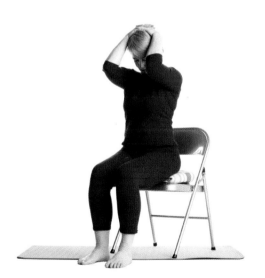

FIGURE 5A
FORWARD-AND-BACK NECK STRETCH, STAGE 1

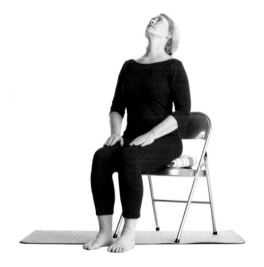

FIGURE 5B
FORWARD-AND-BACK NECK STRETCH, STAGE 2

your ears, so you do not compress the back of your neck. Hold for 3 breaths. Return to Seated Mountain Pose on the exhalation.

Everyday Yoga

When we work at a desk or sit in a chair reading, we often tilt our heads down. To counterbalance that position, do the opposite movement—look up slowly, as in stage 2. Similarly, if you find yourself looking upward for some time, like at the movies, then drop your chin, as in stage 1.

Ear-to-Shoulder Neck Stretch

▼ ▼ ▼ ▼ ▼ ▼ ▼ INCREASES RANGE OF MOTION IN THE SIDES OF THE NECK • RELIEVES NECK TENSION AND PAIN • IMPROVES POSTURE

FOUNDATION: **Pelvis**

PRACTICE WITH CARE: **If you have any diagnosed disk problems in your neck or feel discomfort in this pose, skip it for now, and discuss it with your doctor or therapist.**

PROPS: **1 nonskid mat • 1 chair**

POSSIBLE PROP: **1 blanket or pillow**

This stretch lengthens the sides of your neck. We'll practice it in two stages. Stage 2 provides a deeper stretch.

Stage 1. Begin in Seated Mountain Pose (Figure 1). Sit on a folded blanket or pillow, if you need one. Place your palms on your thighs, relaxed. As you inhale, slowly bring your right ear toward your right shoulder (Figure 6A). Don't strain. On the exhalation, relax both shoulders down from your ears. When you inhale again, feel the lengthening on the left side of your neck, and relax on the exhalation. Hold for 3 breaths, inhale as you return to center, and exhale. Rest here for a few breaths. Then inhale as you move your left ear toward your left shoulder. Hold for 3 breaths. Return to your starting position, finishing in Seated Mountain Pose.

Stage 2. If you are ready for a deeper stretch, after you have brought your right ear toward your right shoulder, lift your right arm and place your right hand on your head a bit above and behind your left ear (Figure 6B). Inhale and feel the lengthening in the left side of your neck. On the exhalation, feel the weight of your hand and arm to help you stretch farther. Hold for 3 breaths. On your last exhalation, return your palm to your thigh. Then inhale your head back to the starting position. Repeat on the other side. Use your breath to help you move slowly. Rest in Seated Mountain Pose.

Everyday Yoga

While talking on the phone or driving with one hand high on the steering wheel, we often tilt our heads to one side or lift one shoulder, while tensing one side of the neck. This neck stretch will help realign your neck and keep it flexible.

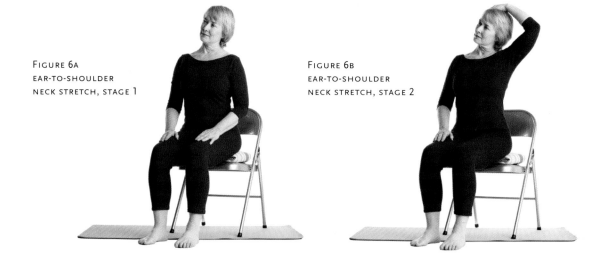

FIGURE 6A
EAR-TO-SHOULDER
NECK STRETCH, STAGE 1

FIGURE 6B
EAR-TO-SHOULDER
NECK STRETCH, STAGE 2

Seated Eagle Pose

GARUDASANA

▼ ▼ ▼ ▼ ▼ ▼ ▼ STRETCHES THE MUSCLES AROUND
THE SHOULDER BLADES AND UPPER BACK • IMPROVES RANGE
OF MOTION IN THE SHOULDERS

FOUNDATION: Pelvis

PROPS: 1 nonskid mat • 1 chair

POSSIBLE PROP: 1 blanket or pillow

Many people have tension in their upper backs, around the shoulder blades, and it can be difficult to figure out how to stretch this area to find relief. Seated Eagle Pose does exactly that. It can provide a wonderful feeling of opening in the upper back and shoulders.

In its classical form, this pose is done while standing with the legs also entwined, but since we are focused primarily on arm and shoulder movements, we'll practice a variation beginning in Seated Mountain Pose (Figure 1). Sit on a folded blanket or pillow, if you need one. Bend your right elbow 90 degrees, with the palm of your right hand facing to the left. Bend your left elbow and place it underneath your right one, crossing your elbows in front of your chest (Figure 7A). If you are unable to cross elbows, place your left hand on the outer side of your right elbow (Figure 7B).

If your elbows are crossed, wrap your left hand around your right forearm, and place the fingers of your left hand on the inside palm of your right hand. Not everyone can cross their arms like this, so if you cannot touch your hands, just move them as far as you can. If your hands are together, move them forward, away from your head. On the inhalation, whatever form you are doing, lift your elbows up as high as they will go without straining, and allow your upper back to widen. On the exhalation, hold the pose and relax your shoulders down from your ears. It is important to keep your neck lengthened. Often, when lifting the arms, we tend to compress the neck, so keep it relaxed. Hold the pose for 3 breaths. On the last exhalation, actively push your elbows down, without collapsing in the chest, and feel the stretch along the tops of your shoulders. Inhale 1 more breath, and release on the exhalation. Rest in Seated Mountain Pose. Repeat on the other side, starting with bending your left elbow 90 degrees. Return to Seated Mountain Pose.

FIGURE 7A
SEATED EAGLE POSE

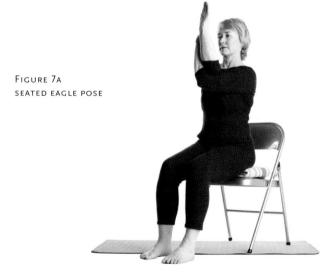

Everyday Yoga

In most of our daily movements, we don't often expand the muscles in the upper back laterally (from the spine out to the sides). And anytime we reach behind to fasten a bra or put something in a rear pocket, we continue to tighten those back muscles. If these activities are difficult for you, try Seated Eagle Pose before doing them. It helps open your upper back and improves the flexibility of your shoulders.

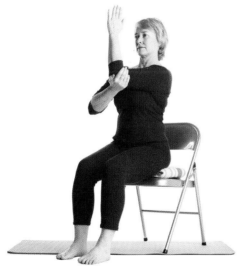

FIGURE 7B
SEATED EAGLE POSE, VARIATION

Prayer Pose

▼ ▼ ▼ ▼ ▼ ▼ STRETCHES THE UNDERSIDES OF THE WRISTS
• OPENS CIRCULATION TO THE HANDS

FOUNDATION: **Pelvis**

PROP: **1 nonskid mat • 1 chair**

POSSIBLE PROP: **1 blanket or pillow**

The loss of flexibility and mobility in your hands and wrists can have a huge impact on your quality of life. Activities such as dressing, cooking, or using a computer keyboard often add tremendous stress to the wrists and can lead to carpal tunnel syndrome, a compression of the nerves in the wrist. Stretches to help open the wrists can be beneficial and should become part of your daily routine.

Begin in Seated Mountain Pose (Figure 1). Sit on a folded blanket or pillow, if you need one. Place your palms together in a prayer position, and hold them about chest level, with your fingers pointed up. Inhale and press the palms together, keeping your shoulders, neck, and jaw relaxed. As you exhale, slowly begin to lower your palms, still keeping them together in Prayer Pose (Figure 8). Your shoulders and upper arms should remain soft and in place, with only the forearms and hands moving down. Inhale again, visualizing the stretch to open the wrists farther. As you exhale, keep your shoulders down from your ears, and move your hands a little lower. Repeat for one more breath, then release and gently shake out your wrists and hands.

Eventually the heels of your hands should be able to move below the level of your elbows, but don't be discouraged if they don't yet. Instead, recognize that this area needs some attention, and remember to practice this stretch often. To keep your wrists balanced and stretched evenly, follow this pose with Reverse Prayer Pose (Figure 9).

Everyday Yoga

Use Prayer Pose before, during, or after activities that stress your hands and wrists— writing, hand sewing and other crafts, cooking, gardening, picking up a baby, working with hand tools, carrying a briefcase or grocery bag, opening drawers—any movements where you are tensing the underside of your wrists.

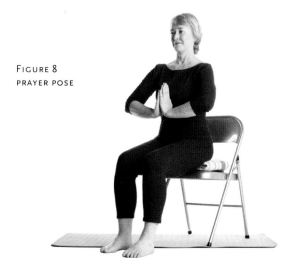

FIGURE 8
PRAYER POSE

Reverse Prayer Pose

VIPARITA NAMASTE

▼ ▼ ▼ ▼ ▼ ▼ ▼ STRETCHES THE TOP PARTS OF THE WRISTS
• INCREASES CIRCULATION TO THE HANDS

FOUNDATION: Pelvis

PROPS: 1 nonskid mat • 1 chair

POSSIBLE PROP: 1 blanket or pillow

It is important to balance your movements, so stretching the outer side, or tops, of your wrists in Reverse Prayer Pose (Figure 9) should always follow Prayer Pose (Figure 8). The tops of your wrists get especially tense when you use a computer keyboard, because you constantly have to flex and hold the wrists up when typing. The same muscles are used when you write or cook. This pose relieves those muscles.

Begin in Seated Mountain Pose (Figure 1). Sit on a folded blanket or pillow, if you need one. Place the backs of your hands together, this time with your fingers pointing down. With an inhalation, press your hands together, keeping them touching all the way up toward the wrists, where they tend to separate. When you exhale, remember to keep your shoulders and upper arms relaxed, while gradually lowering your elbows. Hold the position as you inhale, visualizing the stretch on the tops of your wrists. On the exhalation, try to lower your elbows even farther. Repeat for one more breath, and release and relax. Gently shake out your wrists and hands. In this pose, your elbows should move to a position below the level of your wrists, but if they don't, see what daily practice will bring.

Everyday Yoga

Make this stretch a habit when you get up from your computer or whenever you have been working with your hands. Any time we use our hands to lift or hold, we are tensing the tops of the wrists. Combing or brushing your hair, pulling weeds, stirring a pot on the stove, all add stress to your wrists. Practicing Reverse Prayer Pose after any of these activities will help keep your wrists more supple and pain free.

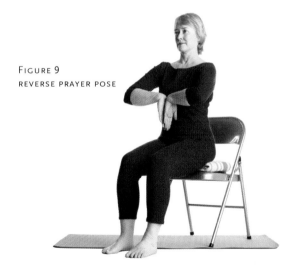

FIGURE 9
REVERSE PRAYER POSE

Cobra Pose

BHUJANGASANA

▼ ▼ ▼ ▼ ▼ ▼ EXPANDS AND LENGTHENS THE MUSCLES
IN THE FRONT OF THE CHEST • LENGTHENS THE SPINE

FOUNDATION: Pelvis

PRACTICE WITH CARE: If you have diagnosed disk problems, consult your doctor
or therapist. If you feel discomfort in your wrists, elbows, or shoulders, try Seated
Cobra Pose instead (Figure 11). Avoid this pose after the first trimester of pregnancy.
If you are a nursing mother and experience discomfort in this pose, move slowly and
stop when necessary.

PROP: 1 nonskid mat

POSSIBLE PROPS: 1 blanket • 1 pillow

Most of our daily tasks require moving the arms forward. We sit at desks, we
drive, we cook, all by reaching to the front. To counter that movement, it is

FIGURE 10A
COBRA POSE

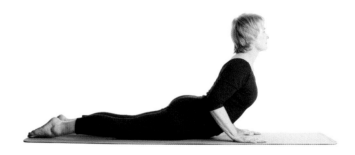

helpful to provide the spine with a pose that uses the opposite movement. Cobra Pose arches the back and opens the chest, with the hands and arms lending support (Figure 10A).

Cobra Pose requires using some arm strength and putting weight on the wrists and hands. If you prefer, you can work from a lower position and rest on your elbows and forearms instead of your hands (Figure 10B). Being on your elbows and forearms puts less stress on the wrists and is easier on the back.

If getting down to the floor is difficult, follow the instructions for getting up and down on page 101. If you do not want to or are unable to work from the floor, practice Seated Cobra Pose instead (Figure 11).

Start by lying on your mat, on your stomach. For comfort, you can lie on a folded blanket on your mat, adding a pillow under your pelvis. Position your hands on the floor along the sides of your chest, so that your fingertips are slightly forward of the tops of your shoulders. (As mentioned, you can be on your elbows and forearms instead of your hands.) Rest your forehead on the floor.

Keep your elbows in by your sides, and press down on your hands (or elbows and forearms). Tighten your buttock muscles to help protect your lower spine, and draw your shoulders down away from your ears. As you inhale, slowly

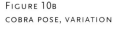
FIGURE 10B
COBRA POSE, VARIATION

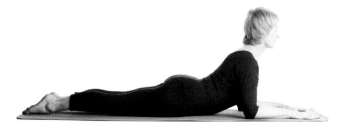

begin to arch your back by lifting your head and then your chest. Visualize the slow, curving motion of a cobra as you arch upward. On the exhalation, focus on relaxing your pelvis.

To avoid tension and compression in the back of your neck, keep your elbows close to the sides of your torso and look straight ahead, not up. How high you lift is not important. Come up only as far as your spine allows, tightening the buttock muscles, lengthening the middle back, and softening the neck.

Inhale, and feel the breath expanding into your chest. On the exhalation, relax into the pose by keeping your shoulders down and your neck, jaw, elbows, and lower back soft. Hold the pose for 3 breaths. On the last exhalation, lower yourself slowly. Relax with your forehead on your mat (or blanket) and your arms back at your sides, or with your forehead on the backs of your folded hands.

Follow this pose with Cat Pose (Figure 12), a countermovement that balances the muscles around the spine by rounding the back.

Everyday Yoga

Any activity where you are rounding your spine forward, such as sitting at a desk, typing, reading, cooking, or gardening, can cause back pain. Practice this back-bending pose before or after these activities to help balance and realign the spine by providing a complementary movement.

Seated Cobra Pose

BHUJANGASANA

▼ ▼ ▼ ▼ ▼ ▼ ▼ EXPANDS THE FRONT OF THE CHEST
• LENGTHENS THE SPINE

FOUNDATION: **Pelvis**

PRACTICE WITH CARE: **If you have diagnosed disk problems or feel discomfort when arching your back, skip this pose for now, and consult your doctor or therapist. Avoid this pose after the first trimester of pregnancy.**

PROPS: **1 nonskid mat • 1 chair**

POSSIBLE PROP: **1 blanket or pillow**

You can practice Seated Cobra Pose (Figure 11) on its own, or as an alternative on those days when Cobra Pose (Figure 10A or Figure 10B) is too strenuous for you. The seated version provides a gentle back arch without adding stress to the wrists or arms.

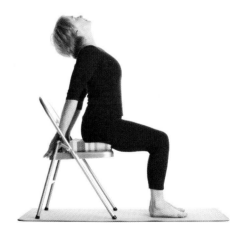

FIGURE 11
SEATED COBRA POSE

Begin in Seated Mountain Pose (Figure 1). Sit on a folded blanket or pillow, if you need one. Bring your arms behind you, and place your hands on the chair seat, with your fingertips facing away from you. If you find it stressful to reach the chair seat, rest your fingertips instead of your palms on the seat.

Inhale, as you lift your ribs and gently arch your middle back. Slowly lift your chin, without compressing the back of your neck. Exhale, and relax your shoulders down from your ears. Visualize your shoulder blades moving down with each exhalation. Soften your eyes and jaw. Hold for 2 more rounds of breath. On the last exhalation, bring your hands back to your thighs, palms down, and let your middle back return to neutral. Drop your chin to your chest for a few breaths, and then rest for a few breaths in Seated Mountain Pose.

Everyday Yoga

Seated Cobra Pose can be done anytime you are in a chair. It provides a feeling of openness in the chest to counter all those forward movements we do in our daily lives. We often round our backs when we bring our arms forward while cooking, writing, typing, reading, carrying groceries, or slouching while watching TV. Take a break and do Seated Cobra Pose before you stand up. You'll be surprised how much better you'll feel.

Cat Pose

BIDALASANA

▽ ▽ ▽ ▽ ▽ ▽ STRETCHES THE MUSCLES ALONG THE SPINE
• RELIEVES TENSION IN THE LOWER BACK AND SHOULDERS
• IMPROVES MOBILITY IN THE PELVIS

FOUNDATION: **Hands and knees**

PRACTICE WITH CARE: **If you have diagnosed disk problems or discomfort when arching your back, move slowly through each stage or practice only stage 2. You may want to consult your doctor or therapist before practicing the pose.**

PROP: **1 nonskid mat**

POSSIBLE PROP: **1 blanket**

We will practice Cat Pose in two stages: first arching your back and then rounding it. In this pose, your hands and knees are your foundation, so take time to firmly establish it. For comfort, you can place a folded blanket on your mat. If getting down to the floor is difficult, follow the instructions in part 3, page 101.

Begin by getting onto your mat, on all fours, with a folded blanket under your hands and feet for comfort, if necessary. Position your hands below your shoulders and your knees apart, below your hips. Distribute your weight throughout your palms and fingers and evenly between your hands and knees.

Look down at your mat, eyes soft, without dropping your head. You will pass through this neutral position as you move back and forth between arching your back and rounding it.

Stage 1. Inhale, and slowly arch your back, as you roll your sitting bones and buttocks up and gently lift your head (Figure 12A). Do not look up. Soften the back of your neck, and relax your jaw. Soften your gaze. You may notice a tendency to push the chin forward as you lift your head, which compresses the back of your neck. So keep your throat soft, as you allow your neck and head to move in a gentle arch.

Stage 2. Exhale, and gently lower your head as you round your middle back and lower your tailbone (Figure 12B). Draw your abdomen in toward your spine. Lift your shoulders away from your hands. Feel the openness in your back and shoulders.

FIGURE 12A
CAT POSE, STAGE 1

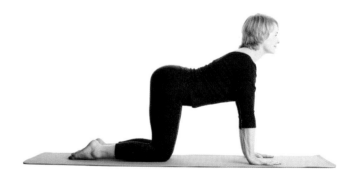

Repeat this sequence 3 times, relying on your slow, gentle inhalations and exhalations to lead you. Rest in the neutral starting position.

Everyday Yoga

Practice Cat Pose in the morning to wake up your back, or before you go to sleep to help relieve any built-up back tension before lying down. When you have had a stressful day, or if you have lower back pain from poor posture or inactivity, this pose is a good one to add to your daily routine.

FIGURE 12B
CAT POSE, STAGE 2

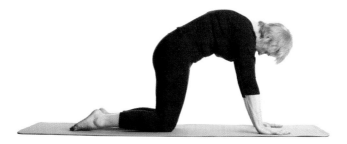

Downward-Facing Dog Pose

ADHO MUKHA SVANASANA

▼ ▼ ▼ ▼ ▼ ▼ ▼ STRETCHES THE BACKS OF THE THIGHS AND CALVES • LENGTHENS THE SPINE • OPENS THE SHOULDERS • STRENGTHENS THE ARMS AND WRISTS • HELPS REDUCE FATIGUE

FOUNDATION: **Hands and feet**

PRACTICE WITH CARE: **If you are in the third trimester of pregnancy, if you are menstruating, or if you have glaucoma, retinal problems, a hiatal hernia, or wrist problems, practice Half Dog Pose instead (Figure 14).**

PROP: **1 nonskid mat**

Downward-Facing Dog Pose (Figure 13) is a wonderful way to bring energy while stretching your arms and legs and lengthening your spine. If you don't want to get down on the floor, then practice Half Dog Pose (Figure 14 A or Figure 14B or Figure 14C).

Begin on all fours on your mat, with your hands directly below your shoulders and your knees hip-width apart. Inhale as you turn your toes under. On the exhalation, lift your knees and hips, and let your head drop gently; look down. On the next inhalation, press down with your hands, drawing your shoulders up and away from your hands, as you lengthen your spine. Do not lock your knees or elbows. If either feels stressed, bend them slightly and then extend them again.

On the next exhalation, keep your back and pelvis stable as you lower your heels toward the floor. If your hamstrings (the muscles along the backs of your thighs) are tight, you may tend to tilt your pelvis when lowering your heels, so only lower them as far as a your lengthened spine allows. With practice, your stretches will improve.

Hold the pose for 3 more even breaths. Focus on lengthening when you inhale and feeling your foundation when you exhale. If you need to come down sooner, then do. You are the best judge of what is right for you. On the last exhalation, lower yourself back to the starting position on your knees. Sit to one side, and gently shake out your hands before standing up.

Everyday Yoga

When you are sedentary or feeling fatigued, Downward-Facing Dog Pose can give you energy. If your legs have been in one position for a while, such as when seated at a desk, the pose will provide a balanced stretch for the backs of your legs and will improve circulation. It also helps maintain strength in your arms, so you can more easily carry bags and push yourself up from a chair. It is one of my favorite everyday poses.

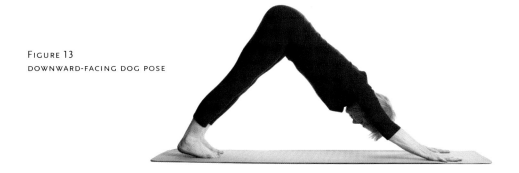

FIGURE 13
DOWNWARD-FACING DOG POSE

Half Dog Pose

ARDHA ADHO MUKHA SVANASANA

▼ ▼ ▼ ▼ ▼ ▼ ▼ STRETCHES THE BACKS OF THE
THIGHS AND CALVES • LENGTHENS THE SPINE •
OPENS THE SHOULDERS • REDUCES FATIGUE

FOUNDATION: Hands and feet

PROPS: 1 nonskid mat • 1 chair

POSSIBLE PROP: 1 towel • a wall

Half Dog Pose can be practiced on its own or as an alternative to Downward-Facing Dog Pose (Figure 13). We will practice this pose in two stages; stage 1 offers two ways of working.

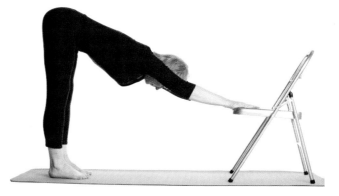

FIGURE 14A
HALF DOG POSE, STAGE 1

Stage 1. Place a chair on your mat, with the seat facing you. Stand in Mountain Pose (Figure 3A). When you feel centered, bend at the hips, and put your hands on the front edge of the seat, shoulder-width apart. Step back with both feet until your hips make an angle a little larger than a right angle (Figure 14A). Draw your hips back from your hands. This lengthens your spine and opens your shoulders. Keep your neck and throat relaxed by looking down. Hold for 3 breaths, focusing on lengthening the spine when you inhale and relaxing into the pose, feeling weight in your hands and feet when you exhale.

Stage 1, alternative. If the stretch using the chair is too intense, practice at a wall. Position the short end of your mat against the wall. Stand in Mountain Pose, facing the wall. Place your hands on the wall at shoulder height, shoulder-width apart. Step back until your torso is parallel to the floor (Figure 14B). Hold for 3 breaths.

To come out of either variation, walk your feet forward, and inhale as you come up to Mountain Pose. Sit down and rest in Seated Mountain Pose (Figure 1).

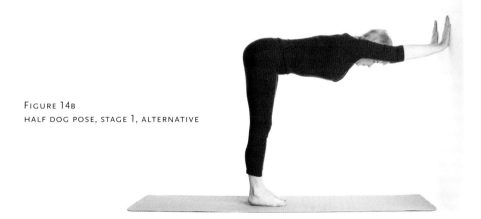

FIGURE 14B
HALF DOG POSE, STAGE 1, ALTERNATIVE

Stage 2. Position a rolled towel so you can move it with your feet. Whether you are using the chair or a wall, to get a deeper stretch in your calves, place the towel so it is under the balls of your feet (Figure 14C). You may need to experiment to get the correct position and size of roll for you. Inhale, lengthen the spine, and draw the hips away from your hands. Exhale, press your heels down, and relax in the pose, feeling weight in your heels. Hold this pose for 3 breaths. On the last exhalation, walk your feet forward, sit down, and rest in Seated Mountain Pose.

Everyday Yoga

Half Dog Pose provides stretches in many areas of the body while also energizing you. When you feel sluggish, this is a wonderful pose to pep you up. If the backs of your legs feel tight from too much walking, standing, or sitting, this pose will help relieve the tension there.

FIGURE 14C
HALF DOG POSE, STAGE 2

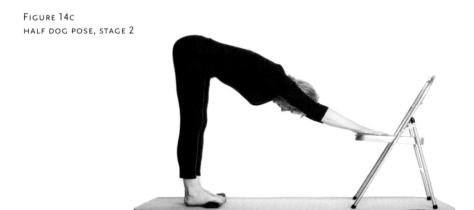

Reclining Hamstring Stretch Pose

SUPTA PADANGUSTHASANA

▼ ▼ ▼ ▼ ▼ ▼ ▼ LENGTHENS THE BACKS OF THE THIGHS
AND CALVES • RELEASES THE PELVIS

FOUNDATION: Pelvis, shoulders, and head

PRACTICE WITH CARE: Avoid this pose if you have sciatica, an injured hamstring, or are in the second half of pregnancy.

PROPS: 1 nonskid mat • 1 strap

POSSIBLE PROPS: 1 blanket • 1 pillow or towel

The hamstrings are a group of three large muscles that run down the back of each thigh. They are attached to the pelvis at the sitting bones, and they influence the tilt, or position, of the pelvis when they are tight. The tilt of the pelvis, in turn, affects the alignment of the spine and, therefore, your posture. Tight hamstrings cause the pelvis to tilt by pulling it down in back, which often leads to lower back pain.

In our daily lives, we are always tightening the hamstring muscles. If you sit a lot, these muscles tighten, because the knees are bent. If you do a lot of exercise, they tighten from the activity. The hamstrings do not get fully stretched during our daily activities, so they must be consciously stretched.

If getting down to the floor is difficult, follow the instructions in part 3, page 101.

Begin Reclining Hamstring Stretch Pose (Figure 15A) by lying on your back on your mat with your strap nearby. If needed, add a folded blanket on top of your mat for a softer surface and a pillow or folded towel behind your head for support.

Bend your right knee, and bring it toward your chest. Keep your tailbone and the back of your left thigh on the floor. This helps align your pelvis while stretching and protects your lower back. If you cannot keep your tailbone and left thigh down, then work with your left leg bent and your foot on the floor, to help keep the tailbone down (Figure 15B)

Wrap the strap around the ball of your right foot. Hold one end of the strap in each hand, and gradually straighten the leg. Work your hands up the strap until your arms are straight and hanging from the strap, so your shoulders can relax. Resist the tendency to grip the strap and tense the shoulders; keep the hands and shoulders soft.

You might be tempted to allow the pelvis to tilt as you draw your extended leg toward you with the strap, thinking you are pulling the leg closer to you

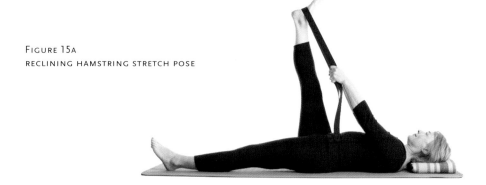

FIGURE 15A
RECLINING HAMSTRING STRETCH POSE

and getting a better stretch, but this only stretches your lower back. So keep your tailbone on the floor.

Use your breath to help you concentrate. As you follow the stretch, lengthen with each inhalation, visualizing the stretch moving up the back of your leg toward your foot. With every exhalation, hold the pose, relax, and soften the leg muscles, shoulders, and pelvis. Follow the stretch down the back of your leg toward your sitting bones as you exhale.

Hold the pose for 5 full, slow rounds of breath. Then release the strap, draw your leg into your chest, and return to the starting position. Repeat on the other side. You may find that you need to practice with the down leg extended on one side but in a bent position on the other side.

Everyday Yoga

You can practice Reclining Hamstring Stretch Pose in the morning, to wake up your legs, or before you go to bed, to relax them. You might try it in lieu of Downward-Facing Dog Pose (Figure 13) when it is hot or you are tired, or when you are practicing in the evening and want a less invigorating practice. You can also practice it before Downward-Facing Dog Pose.

FIGURE 15B
RECLINING HAMSTRING STRETCH POSE, VARIATION

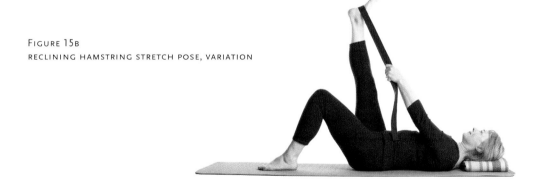

Seated Hamstring Stretch Pose

PADANGUSTHASANA

▼ ▼ ▼ ▼ ▼ ▼ ▼ LENGTHENS THE BACKS OF THE THIGHS
AND CALVES • RELEASES THE PELVIS

FOUNDATION: Pelvis

PRACTICE WITH CARE: Skip this pose if you have sciatica or an injured hamstring.

PROPS: 1 nonskid mat • 1 chair

POSSIBLE PROP: 1 blanket or pillow

A few words about moving forward while in a chair: In Seated Hamstring Stretch Pose (Figure 16), you will be moving forward from the hips. To learn where this point is, place your thumbs in the crease where your thighs meet your torso. This is where your movement will originate. Make sure your foundation is stable on the chair as you move forward.

Begin in Seated Mountain Pose (Figure 1). Sit on a folded blanket or pillow, if you need one. Take the time to feel balanced before moving forward. Feel your sitting bones in contact with the chair seat and your feet in contact with the floor. Extend your right leg out in front of you. Place your heel on the floor, toes pointing toward the ceiling.

Inhale, lift your chest, and lengthen your spine, as you slowly lower your torso forward, moving the right and left sides of the rib cage evenly. Place your left forearm or hand on your left thigh, near your knee, and your right hand on your right thigh. Make sure you are not leaning toward the left leg. If you are, adjust your position so that your breastbone is centered between your legs.

Exhale, soften the abdomen, and relax your shoulders. You should feel a pleasant stretch in the back of your right thigh. The more you flex your foot, the more you will feel the stretch in your right calf. Hold this pose for 5 full, slow breaths. Sit up slowly, and return to Seated Mountain Pose. Repeat on the other side.

Everyday Yoga

Practice Seated Hamstring Stretch Pose anytime your legs feel tense or before standing up if you have been sitting for a long time. Your legs will always appreciate this stretch.

FIGURE 16
SEATED HAMSTRING STRETCH POSE

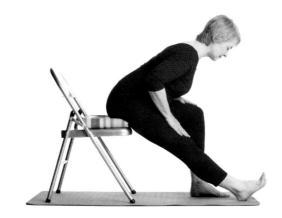

Reclining Twist Pose

JATHARA PARIVARTANASANA

▼ ▼ ▼ ▼ ▼ ▼ ▼ ROTATES THE SPINE • OPENS THE CHEST
• RELIEVES BACK PAIN

FOUNDATION: Pelvis and shoulders

PRACTICE WITH CARE: If you have diagnosed disk problems in your lower back or feel discomfort in the pose, move carefully, or skip the pose and consult your doctor or therapist.

PROP: 1 nonskid mat

POSSIBLE PROPS: 2 blankets • 1 pillow or towel

The Chinese have a saying: "To move is to live." The more we keep active, within our abilities, the better our quality of life will be. So make it a priority to keep your spine as flexible as possible.

Reclining Twist Pose (Figure 17) rotates the spine in a twisting motion and also opens the chest. If getting down to the floor is difficult but you want to try this pose, follow the instructions for getting up and down in part 3, page 101. If you don't want to get down on the floor, practice Seated Twist Pose instead (Figure 18A or Figure 18B).

Lie on your back on your mat. For comfort, you can add a folded blanket on top of your mat and a pillow or folded towel under your neck. Take several breaths to settle in. Feel the backs of your calves and thighs in contact with the floor. Soften the area around your navel.

Bend your right knee, and draw it toward your chest, keeping your left leg extended. Place your left hand on the outside of your right knee and your right arm out to the side, on the floor, at shoulder level, with the palm up. Inhale, and on the exhalation roll your right knee as far to the left as possible, while both shoulders remain on the floor. If your knee does not touch the floor or if you feel strain holding it in this position, then rest it on a folded or rolled blanket. (Experiment with the blanket height until you are comfortable.) With an exhalation, turn your head gently to the right, being careful not to strain your neck, and soften the muscles around your abdomen.

When you inhale, let your breath expand your chest, so that your ribs lift slightly toward the right. Feel the stretch through your fingers instead of stopping the stretch at the wrist. Lengthen all the way out to your fingertips, sensing the energy flow. On the exhalation, be aware of your shoulders in contact with the floor. Soften your abdomen, throat, and jaw. Relax your forehead, and feel the weight of your right leg move toward the left, as you twist. Hold this pose for 3 breaths.

FIGURE 17
RECLINING TWIST POSE

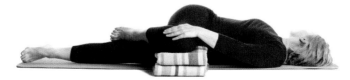

Inhale, and gently lift your right leg back to center. Exhale, and extend it back to the floor. Rest until you feel ready to repeat on the other side.

Everyday Yoga

If you have lower back pain from poor posture or from being sedentary (and not from diagnosed disk problems), or if you feel fatigued, do Reclining Twist Pose to relieve tension and provide energy. Practice it as a stress break during the day.

Seated Twist Pose

▼ ▼ ▼ ▼ ▼ ▼ ▼ ROTATES THE SPINE • OPENS THE CHEST •
RELIEVES GENERAL BACK PAIN

FOUNDATION: Pelvis

PRACTICE WITH CARE: If you have diagnosed disk problems in your lower back or feel discomfort in this pose, move carefully, or skip the pose and consult your doctor or therapist. If you are pregnant, keep the belly soft.

PROPS: 1 nonskid mat • 1 chair

POSSIBLE PROP: 1 blanket or pillow

In Seated Twist Pose, the pelvis remains stable, unlike in the floor variation, Reclining Twist Pose (Figure 17), where the pelvis moves.

Begin in Seated Mountain Pose (Figure 1), using a folded blanket or pillow, if you need one. Take a few breaths to center yourself. Then turn toward the right, and sit sideways on your chair. Sit on the full seat, not just the edge, with your right hip touching the back of the chair. Align your pelvis in Seated Mountain Pose, lengthening the spine and feeling your feet in contact with the floor.

Inhale gently, leading the twist from your navel as you turn toward the right. Let your head and shoulders follow. Keep both knees in the same plane; do not allow your left knee to move forward of the right knee.

You can choose from two hand positions: Reach with your right hand and hold the outer right edge of the chair back and place your left hand on the left edge (Figure 18A). If you can't reach this far, then place your right hand on top of the chair back and your left on the outside of your right thigh, which will give you some leverage as you twist (Figure 18B). Exhale, and relax your shoulders.

Inhale and lengthen your spine, as you lead the twist from the navel. Press your right hand against the chair to enhance the twist. Do not strain your neck. On the inhalation, feel the expansion across your front chest, side ribs, and upper back. Exhale, and relax your shoulders down from your ears. Still exhaling, visualize yourself coiling to the right, allowing your shoulders to follow the

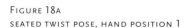

FIGURE 18A
SEATED TWIST POSE, HAND POSITION 1

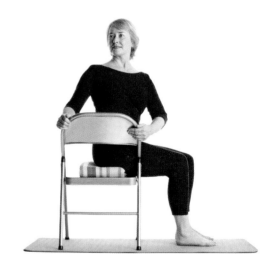

movement of the navel and your neck and head to follow the movement of the shoulders. Relax your eyes and jaw.

Hold for 3 rounds of breaths. On the last exhalation, uncoil and return to Seated Mountain Pose. Rest until you feel centered. Now turn to the other side, and repeat the pose on the left.

Everyday Yoga

I practice Seated Twist Pose often throughout the day when working at my computer. Try it whenever you are in a chair and need a yoga break. You will see how it energizes you!

FIGURE 18B
SEATED TWIST POSE, HAND POSITION 2

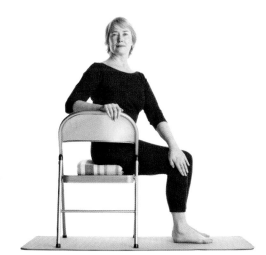

Reclining Thread-the-Needle

▼ ▼ ▼ ▼ ▼ ▼ ▼ REDUCES KNEE STRAIN • INCREASES
HIP MOBILITY • STRETCHES THE BUTTOCKS AND OUTER HIP MUSCLES

FOUNDATION: Pelvis, shoulders, and head

PRACTICE WITH CARE: Work at your comfort level, moving slowly if your hips are
tight and don't allow for much rotation of the top leg.

PROP: 1 nonskid mat

POSSIBLE PROPS: 1 blanket • 1 pillow or towel • 1 strap

Lie on your back on the mat. If you prefer not to get on the floor, practice
Seated Thread-the-Needle (Figure 20). For comfort, you can place a folded
blanket under you and a pillow or folded towel behind your head. Take time
to settle in, feeling the contact of your body against your mat.

FIGURE 19A
RECLINING THREAD-THE-NEEDLE

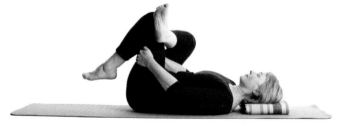

To begin Reclining Thread-the-Needle, bend your knees, placing your feet on the floor near your buttocks. Lift your right leg, and place your right ankle on your left thigh, above the knee. Keep your right foot flexed, with your heel moving away from your right knee and your toes pointing toward the ceiling. Lift your left foot off the floor, and draw your leg toward your chest. As you do, keep your sacrum (the area above the tailbone and below the waist) on the floor. Grasp behind the left thigh with both hands, drawing your leg closer to your chest (Figure 19A). If you cannot reach behind your thigh, place a strap around the back of your thigh, and hold the strap with both hands (Figure 19B). Notice the stretch in your right buttock and outer right hip.

You may feel a tendency to roll back and tilt the pelvis when lifting the leg, which can stress the lower back. In this pose, your pelvis is part of your foundation; it should not roll back. You can feel the correct pelvic position by keeping the weight off your waistline in the back and feeling more weight in the areas above and below the waist. Inhale, and let the breath expand your chest as you stretch the back of your right thigh. Exhale, relax your shoulders and abdomen, and soften the muscles in your hips. Hold the pose for 3 breaths. On the last

FIGURE 19B
RECLINING THREAD-THE-NEEDLE, VARIATION

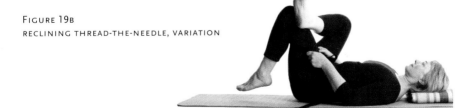

exhalation, lower your left foot to the floor, unbend the right leg, and release the right foot to the floor. Then extend both legs. Take a few rounds of breath to center yourself. Then repeat the sequence on the other side, crossing the left foot above the right knee.

After completing each side, rest with both legs extended for a few rounds of breath before standing up.

Everyday Yoga

Walking, gardening, or sitting for long periods can tighten the muscles on the backs of your legs and hips. Practice Reclining Thread-the-Needle to open your hips and release tension from the hamstrings (the muscles that go from the backs of your legs into your buttocks).

Seated Thread-the-Needle

▼ ▼ ▼ ▼ ▼ ▼ ▼ REDUCES KNEE STRAIN • INCREASES HIP
FLEXIBILITY • STRETCHES THE MUSCLES AROUND THE BUTTOCKS
AND OUTER HIPS • RELIEVES BACK TENSION

FOUNDATION: Pelvis

PRACTICE WITH CARE: Work at your comfort level,
moving slowly to protect the knee if your hips are tight
and don't allow for much rotation in the top leg.

PROPS: 1 nonskid mat • 1 chair

POSSIBLE PROP: 1 blanket or pillow

You can practice Seated Thread-the-Needle
(Figure 20) in its own right or as an alternative to Reclining Thread-the-Needle (Figure 19A or Figure 19B).

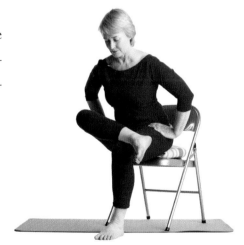

FIGURE 20
SEATED THREAD-THE-NEEDLE

Place your chair at the long edge of your mat. Begin in Seated Mountain Pose (Figure 1). Lift your right leg, and place your right ankle onto your left thigh, a few inches above the knee, with your right knee moving out to the right. Keep the right foot flexed. Place your fingers at your hip creases and your thumbs on your hips.

As you inhale, lengthen your spine to sit up tall. As you exhale, slowly lean forward, leading with the navel and sternum, keeping the head and neck relaxed. Do not lead with your chin, as that compresses the back of your neck.

With each inhalation, concentrate on lengthening the spine and stretching the back of the right thigh. With each exhalation, relax your shoulders and abdomen, softening the muscles in your hip sockets. Hold the pose for 3 breaths. On your next inhalation, leading with your sternum, sit up. Grasp under your right knee with your right hand to release your right leg, and lower it to the floor. Rest in Seated Mountain Pose until you are ready to repeat the sequence on the left side. When you finish the second side, come back to Seated Mountain Pose.

Everyday Yoga

Practice this exercise while sitting at your desk or in any seated position. It will help keep your hips and the backs of your thighs more flexible. After walking, climbing stairs, or doing housework, this pose helps soften the muscles that become tense from use.

Dancer Pose

NATARAJASANA

▼ ▼ ▼ ▼ ▼ ▼ ▼ STRETCHES THE FRONT THIGHS
• OPENS THE SHOULDERS • IMPROVES BALANCE AND POSTURE

FOUNDATION: Feet and pelvis

PRACTICE WITH CARE: If you have diagnosed disk problems
in your lower back, practice Side-Lying Dancer Pose instead.

PROPS: 1 nonskid mat • 1 chair or a wall

POSSIBLE PROPS: 1 strap

The muscles in the front thighs contract when we sit, walk, and exercise. This leads to tight thigh muscles, which can influence the position of the pelvis, affecting posture and contributing to lower back pain. Dancer Pose gives us a way to stretch these muscles. We will practice this pose in two stages.

Stage 1. Stand on your mat in Mountain Pose (Figure 3), with a chair or wall in front of you for balance. Hold on to the top of the chair back (or the wall) with your left hand, and bend your right knee. Reach around behind you with your right hand, and take hold of your right foot or ankle (Figure 21A). If you cannot reach your foot without twisting your back and neck, wrap a strap around your ankle and hold both ends with your right hand (Figure 21B). If this is difficult, try Side-Lying Dancer Pose (Figure 22) instead.

Do not lift your right hip or arch your lower back when you lift the foot. Instead, focus on your left foot, which is your foundation, along with your pelvis; both should remain stable, as in Mountain Pose. Inhale, and lift your side ribs. Exhale, and lengthen through the front right thigh, from the hip down to the knee. Hold the pose for 3 rounds of breath. On the last exhalation, release your foot (or ankle) and lower your foot to the floor. Stand in Mountain Pose. Then repeat the sequence on the other side.

Stage 2. This stage improves balance and stretches the thigh. When you feel ready to challenge yourself, take your left hand away from the support, and lift your arm overhead, palm facing to the right (Figure 21C). To help you remain

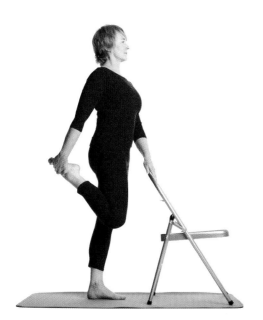
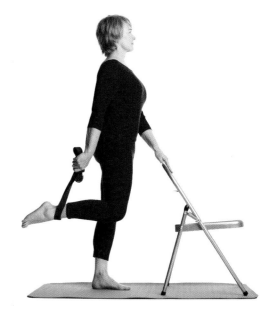

stable, do not lift your shoulders when you lift your arm. Drop your shoulders down from your ears. Keep your jaw relaxed and your eyes soft, focused on one spot for easier balance. Hold this position for 3 breaths. On your last exhalation, lower your arm back to the chair (or wall) for support, as you release your right leg and lower it to Mountain Pose. Repeat on the left side. End in Mountain Pose.

Everyday Yoga

Practice Dancer Pose after sitting, climbing stairs, or gardening, to release built-up tension from flexing the hips.

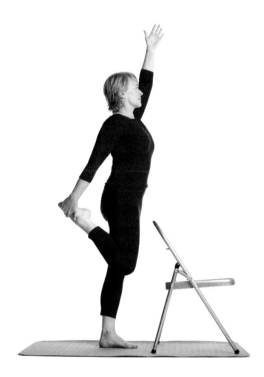

LEFT TO RIGHT:

FIGURE 21A
DANCER POSE, STAGE 1

FIGURE 21B
DANCER POSE, STAGE 1, VARIATION

FIGURE 21C
DANCER POSE, STAGE 2

Side-Lying Dancer Pose

NATARAJASANA

▼ ▼ ▼ ▼ ▼ ▼ ▼ STRETCHES THE FRONTS OF
THE THIGHS • OPENS THE SHOULDERS

FOUNDATION: Pelvis

PRACTICE WITH CARE: If you experience pain or discomfort when you reach
behind and take hold of your foot in Dancer Pose (Figure 21A or Figure 21B),
then practice Side-Lying Dancer Pose (Figure 22) instead. If getting down to
the floor is difficult, follow the instructions in part 3, page 101.

PROP: 1 nonskid mat

POSSIBLE PROPS: 1 blanket • 1 pillow or towel

Start by lying on your mat on your back. For more comfort, you can add a
blanket to soften the mat surface. Take time to center yourself. When you feel
ready, roll onto your left side. You have two choices for positioning your head
and arms: either rest your head on your raised left arm, or place your left arm
out to the front, palm down, and rest your head on a pillow or folded towel.
Whatever position you chose, keep your throat soft and neck relaxed.

Try to keep your legs together as you bend both knees. Without twisting,
grasp your right foot or ankle with your right hand. Inhale, and stretch your
right thigh muscles by lengthening the knee away from the shoulders. Exhale,

and relax and soften the muscles in your hips and thighs. Hold the pose for 3 breaths. On the last exhalation, release your foot, and roll onto your back. When you feel ready, roll onto your right side and repeat the sequence. When done, lie on your back for a few breaths before getting up.

Everyday Yoga

As with Dancer Pose, this is a good stretch to practice after sitting, climbing stairs, or gardening.

FIGURE 22
SIDE-LYING DANCER POSE

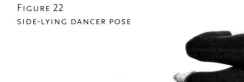

Legs-Up-the-Wall Pose

VIPARITA KARANI

▼ ▼ ▼ ▼ ▼ ▼ ▼ REDUCES FATIGUE • LOWERS BLOOD
PRESSURE • REDUCES SWELLING IN THE LOWER LEGS

FOUNDATION: Pelvis, shoulders, and head

PRACTICE WITH CARE: Avoid this pose if you are menstruating or past the first trimester of pregnancy, or if you have sciatica or a hiatal hernia. Consult with your doctor or therapist if you have concerns about elevating your legs.

PROP: 1 nonskid mat • a wall

POSSIBLE PROPS: 1 pillow or towel • 2 blankets

When you don't want to exercise but your legs feel tired, this pose can provide you with a feeling of lightness and give you energy. It improves the circulation in your legs and provides an alternative to Relaxation Pose (Figure 24). If getting down on the floor is difficult, follow the instructions in part 3, page 101.

Begin Legs-Up-the-Wall Pose (Figure 23) by placing your mat perpendicular to the wall. Sit sideways, with your hips about 8 to 10 inches from the wall. Then swing around so your legs move up the wall and you are lying on your back. Place your head on a pillow or folded towel to keep your neck relaxed; adjust it as needed. For more comfort, you can add a folded blanket under your lower back and hips. Place it so that your sacrum rests on the blanket but your tailbone hangs over the edge. You can add another blanket lengthwise to support your back and head, instead of a pillow or folded towel for just your head.

On each inhalation, visualize energy going up your legs to your feet. On each exhalation, let your hips and pelvis and your head and shoulders relax and feel heavy. Stay in the pose for as long as you feel comfortable, but not longer than 20 minutes. Come out if your feet begin to tingle. Before standing up, bring your knees to your chest, and gently roll to one side for a few breaths. Move slowly.

Everyday Yoga

Legs-Up-the-Wall Pose is great to practice after a long day of being on your feet. It is also helpful to bring circulation back to swollen or cramped legs after traveling on an airplane. I like to practice it in the evening because it makes my legs feel lighter and less tired before I go to sleep.

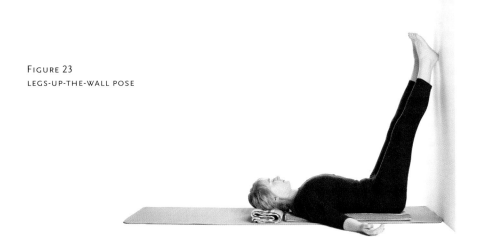

FIGURE 23
LEGS-UP-THE-WALL POSE

Relaxation Pose

SAVASANA

▼ ▼ ▼ ▼ ▼ ▼ ▼ RELEASES MUSCLE TENSION
• REDUCES STRESS AND FATIGUE

FOUNDATION: Pelvis, shoulder, head

PRACTICE WITH CARE: If you are pregnant, practice Side-Lying Relaxation Pose (Figure 26) instead. If you have a cold or difficulty breathing easily, skip this pose.

PROP: 1 nonskid mat

POSSIBLE PROPS: 2 blankets • 1 pillow

Give yourself the gift of relaxation every day. You will be amazed how stopping and quieting your body and mind can release tension, reduce stress, and give you energy.

We will practice Relaxation Pose (Figure 24), with a guided body visualization. If you prefer to practice a guided visualization from one of the other relaxation poses or from part 3, feel free to do so.

To begin, lie on your back on your mat (or on a carpeted floor). If lying on the floor is uncomfortable for your back, try Relaxation Pose with Chair (Figure 25) instead. If getting down to the floor is difficult, follow the instructions in part 3, page 101. For comfort, you can place a folded blanket on your mat and a pillow under your head (or under your neck and head). If you tend to get chilly, cover up with a blanket. You might ask someone to read the following instructions to you or tape yourself reading them so you can relax more easily.

Place your feet hip-width apart and yours arms by the sides of your torso. We'll move throughout the body, first contracting then releasing the muscles, so you learn to feel the difference between tension and relaxation.

Lift your right leg a few inches, point your toes, then push your heel forward, and gently lower the leg. Repeat on the left side: lift the leg, point the toes, flex the foot, and lower it back down. Let both feet completely relax and flop open. Lift your hips, draw your tailbone toward the ceiling, and lower back down. Leave your head on the floor as you lift your chest and shoulders, roll your shoulders back and down, and then lower them.

Lift your right arm a few inches, make a fist and tense it, then stretch your fingers out, turn your whole arm so your palm faces the ceiling, and lower the arm. It should be about 12 inches from your hips. Repeat on the left side: lift the arm, make a fist and tense it, stretch the fingers open, turn the whole arm so the palm is up, and lower it back down.

FIGURE 24
RELAXATION POSE

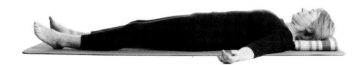

Now roll your head slowly from one side to the other and back to the center. Do you notice any residual tension in your body? Where is it? Inhale all the tension up into your face. Squeeze your eyes shut, scrunch your lips, and tighten your facial muscles. Then open your eyes and, with your mouth wide, stick out your tongue. Then let your face settle into relaxation, as you close your eyes and mouth. Inhale slowly, and on the exhalation let out a long, audible AAAHHH.

Guided Body Visualization. Begin by imagining a warm feeling starting at the tips of your toes, flowing up to your heels, then to the backs of your ankles, and up to your calves. Let your calves feel soft and relaxed. Then move up the backs of your knees, to the backs of your thighs. Let the backs of both legs feel long and warm and relaxed. Now move the warmth around to the tops of your thighs and soften them, so both legs feel completely relaxed and heavy. Follow the warm flow up into your hips. Let your hips relax: make them feel heavy, sinking into the floor.

Next, move the warm flow to the base of your spine, and feel the warmth spread across your lower back. (Do not push the small of your back into the floor. Your lower back has a natural arch that should remain.) Move the warm flow up your spine, and feel it spread across the middle part of your back. Concentrate on keeping your back soft, warm, and relaxed. Continue to the upper part of your back, so your whole back feels relaxed and heavy. Move the focus to your shoulders, and let the muscles of your shoulders relax. Let them drop, so your back and shoulders are soft and heavy, sinking into the floor.

Follow the warmth down your arms, from the upper part of your arms to your elbows, to your forearms, and down to your wrists. Then focus on bringing warmth to the palms of your hands, and feel it spread to your fingers. Let any tension in your body flow out your fingertips, so your hands feel light and your arms, heavy and relaxed.

Now bring the warmth from your shoulders up into your neck. Swallow and soften your throat. Move the warmth around to the back of your neck, and let your neck feel long and relaxed. Follow the warmth from the back of your neck to the back of your head, up to the top of your head, and around to your forehead.

Soften your eyebrows, and smooth out the lines from your forehead. Relax your eyelids, allowing your eyeballs to feel heavy and sink in their sockets. Relax your ears; listen inside to the sound of your heartbeat and your breathing. Relax your nose; feel the movement of air in and out with every breath. Now relax your mouth. Let your tongue rest in your mouth and your jaw relax.

Now move inside, down your throat into your lungs. Watch as they expand with every inhalation, and follow them as they contract when you exhale. Breathe slowly, keeping your lungs relaxed.

All your inner organs feel warm, soft, and relaxed: your kidneys, your liver, your intestines, and your stomach. Now focus on your heart. Breathe slowly, in and out, to the sound of your heartbeat, and relax.

Stay in the pose as long as you want. To come out, bend one knee at a time, and roll onto your right side. Remain there for a few breaths, and then use your arms to help you sit up.

Everyday Yoga

If you are unable to get down to and up from the floor, practice on your bed. You can use Relaxation Pose to help you fall asleep or to rest deeply on those nights when you can't fall asleep or stay asleep. I recommend that you take a relaxation break every afternoon! To vary your practice, you can alternate Relaxation Pose with Relaxation Pose with Chair (Figure 25) or Side-Lying Relaxation Pose (Figure 26), doing a different variation each day or at different times of day. Let "do more of less" be a guide for your life!

Relaxation Pose with Chair

SAVASANA

▼ ▼ ▼ ▼ ▼ ▼ RELEASES MUSCLE TENSION • REDUCES STRESS
AND FATIGUE • SOOTHES LOWER BACK DISCOMFORT

FOUNDATION: Pelvis, shoulders, and head

PRACTICE WITH CARE: If you are pregnant, practice Side-Lying Relaxation Pose (Figure 26). If you have a cold or difficulty breathing easily, skip this pose.

PROPS: 1 nonskid mat • 1 chair

POSSIBLE PROPS: 2 blankets • 1 pillow or towel

If you have lower back discomfort, Relaxation Pose with Chair (Figure 25) will be soothing. You can also try Side-Lying Relaxation Pose (Figure 26) as an alternative.

FIGURE 25
RELAXATION POSE WITH CHAIR

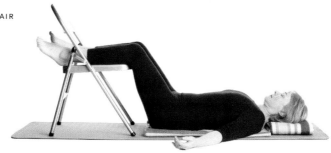

Ask someone to read the instructions to you, or tape yourself reading them, so you can relax more easily. My students with fibromyalgia often want to focus on areas other than their bodies when relaxing. This color visualization provides a wonderful and healing way to do that. Colors have been shown to influence us in many ways, both physically and mentally. They can evoke memories or emotions, and so the following visualization might offer some helpful and surprising avenues to help you relax. Let your responses to my suggestions be spontaneous. Some may appear as images, while others may come as emotions or sensations. If you prefer, you can select a guided visualization from one of the other relaxation poses or from part 3.

To begin, place a chair on your mat (or on a carpeted floor) and lie down on your back in front of it. If getting down to the floor is difficult, follow the instructions in part 3, page 101. For comfort, you can add a folded blanket on your mat and a pillow under your head (or under your head and neck). Place your legs on the chair at about a 90-degree angle to your hips. If you are chilly, cover up with a blanket. Let your legs relax, feet slightly apart and flopped out, and bring your arms comfortably away from your sides, with palms facing up.

Guided Color Visualization. Take the next few minutes to settle into the pose. With each exhalation, let your body feel heavy, relaxed, and still. Begin by focusing your senses on the color red. Can you see red? This color can evoke feelings of anger or anxiety or sensations of pain. Or maybe you can feel red heat from glowing embers. What is the sound of red? Do you hear clashing drums? What comes to you when you smell red? Maybe it's a red rose. Whatever appears, smell the red. What does red taste like? Cherries or tomatoes?

Focus on whatever comes, and taste red. What does red feel like? Roll around in red. Breathe, and let your senses experience red.

Now watch as the red melts into orange. Discover orange. Can you see it? Perhaps you remember a glorious sunset. Maybe orange brings feelings of warmth and security. Can you hear the sound of orange in a cello's low notes? When you sense the taste and smell of orange, maybe you visualize the fruit. Or maybe you see carrots. Let your mind and senses roam around and discover orange. What does orange feel like? Let your skin sense it. Breathe orange.

Then watch as the orange transforms into yellow. Yellow can create feelings of happiness and joy. Or maybe yellow is corn or sunshine. What does yellow sound like? What does it taste like? Smell like? Immerse yourself in yellow. Breathe yellow.

Yellow slowly changes to green. How do you experience green? Green can be a sensation of abundance. Perhaps it appears as an expansive grassy meadow. Maybe you taste green peppers. Or you might taste and smell the essence of limes. Can you hear the sound of green in the wind through the trees? Feel the sensation of green on your skin. Breathe green.

Watch as green slowly becomes blue. With blue may come a feeling of peaceful calm. Maybe blue is an open sky, where you can soar. Or blue might be a vast ocean, where you are floating freely. What does blue sound like? Perhaps it is the water lapping against the shore. What does blue taste like? Blueberries? What does blue feel like? A soft breeze? Rest in blue. Enjoy the experience of blue. Breathe blue.

Blue turns into purple. Visualize purple. It is magical, mystical, regal. The setting sun casts a purple glow across the sky above and earth below. Can you feel the smooth purple of eggplant or taste the delicious purple of grapes? Do you smell the delicate purple of lilacs? However purple comes to you, let your senses experience purple. Breathe purple.

And now, the purple fades, and everything around you becomes white. White can be a feeling of energy, or white light, or purity. Feel whiteness on your skin, and then breathe gentle rays of white light into your lungs, until they feel full. With each exhalation, let the white light stream from your lungs down into your body, and watch as it moves into your torso, then into your hips, down the tops of your thighs, to your knees, your shins, and all the way to your ankles. Keep breathing and filling your body with white light, as it moves from your ankles into the tops of your feet, to your toes, and into the bottoms of your feet.

Then let it move up and fill the back of your body: up your calves, the backs of your knees, to the backs of your thighs. Then sense it in your buttocks, your lower back, your middle back, your upper back, and your shoulders. Now watch as this light moves down your outer arms to your elbows, to your forearms, and to your wrists. Feel the energy in your fingers, then your palms, the undersides of your wrists, your inner forearms, your upper arms, and back to your shoulders.

So now your entire body—from your shoulders down to your toes—is filled with white light. Watch as it moves into your neck, your jaw, to the back of your head, your nose and cheeks, your eyes. Let the light move from your forehead, to the top of your head, filling it. You are filled with white light. Feel its energy alive throughout your body. There are no places left to fill in your body, so the white light begins to emanate from your body. The walls separating the white light inside your body from the white light that surrounds the outside of your body dissolve. What remains is white light and the sound of your heart beating.

Stay in this pose as long as you want. To come out, slowly draw your knees from the chair seat to your chest. Roll to one side, and take a few breaths before sitting up.

Everyday Yoga

You can use Relaxation Pose with Chair whenever you can find the time. It will energize you and help relieve stress from a busy workday. Also, resting your legs on a chair seat will improve circulation after traveling or sitting in one position for a long time. Practice the color visualization in bed to help you fall asleep.

Side-Lying Relaxation Pose
SAVASANA

▼ ▼ ▼ ▼ ▼ ▼ RELEASES MUSCLE TENSION
• REDUCES STRESS AND FATIGUE

FOUNDATION: Pelvis

PROP: 1 nonskid mat • 2 blankets • 2 pillows or towels, or 1 of each

POSSIBLE PROPS: 1 bolster • a wall • 1 blanket

Side-Lying Relaxation Pose (Figure 26) can be practiced instead of Relaxation Pose (Figure 24) or Relaxation Pose with Chair (Figure 25). It offers an alternative for times when you might not feel comfortable lying on your back. It is a wonderful pose to practice during pregnancy.

We will practice Side-Lying Relaxation Pose with guided slow breathing. Most of us only fill the top third of our lungs when we breathe. Slow breathing will help you learn to breathe more fully. This type of breathing is a form of pranayama. It is different from Breathing Awareness (Figure 2A and Figure 2B), in that you consciously use the exhalations to help you focus on relaxing.

For Side-Lying Relaxation Pose, lie on your left side on a mat (or carpeted floor). You can lie on your right side if it is more comfortable. If getting down to the floor is difficult, follow the instructions in part 3, page 101. Place a folded blanket on your mat and a pillow or folded towel under your head to keep your neck relaxed.

Position a folded blanket or pillow between your lower legs to avoid knee strain. Extend your left arm out in front of you, with the palm up. Support your hand on a folded towel. If this position is uncomfortable, then bend your elbow. Rest your right hand gently on your right hip.

Using a bolster (or a rolled blanket) can be comforting. You can either hug it close to the front of your body or place it between your back and a wall. If you tend to get chilly, cover up with a blanket.

Read the instructions until you can remember them before beginning. You can also have someone read this section while you practice or tape yourself reading it, so you can just listen and relax. To vary your practice, you can select a guided visualization from one of the other relaxation poses or from part 3, or listen to your favorite soothing music instead.

Guided Slow Breathing. Take a few minutes to settle into the support of the props. When you feel ready, begin by observing your breath as it enters your nose when you inhale. Feel it move inside, filling your lungs. Can you

FIGURE 26
SIDE-LYING RELAXATION POSE

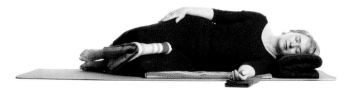

sense where the breath goes and how much breath you have taken in? As you inhale, see if you can breathe deeper, expanding your lungs and drawing the air into all the parts of your lungs: the bottom, the middle, the top. On the exhalation, feel your lungs empty: first from the top, then the middle, then the bottom. Continue for a few rounds of breath, letting tension melt away with each exhalation.

When you feel ready, try making your next inhalation slower and longer. Watch the breath as you fill your lungs. Feel them expand. Then exhale, and let your breath take the tension with it as it leaves you. Continue inhaling slower and deeper with each breath, relaxing and melting the tension from your body with each exhalation. When you have practiced slow breathing long enough, breathe normally and just rest.

You can remain in the pose itself for as long as you like. It is almost impossible to stay too long! When you are ready, open your eyes and, moving slowly, remove the props. Use your arms to help you sit up. Take a few breaths before standing.

Everyday Yoga

To vary your practice, you can alternate this pose with Relaxation Pose (Figure 24) or Relaxation Pose with Chair (Figure 25). Whatever pose you choose, give yourself the gift of relaxation at least once every day: always at the end of your asana or pranayama practice and anytime you need to rest, relax, and restore.

Part III:

Practicing Yoga for Fibromyalgia

▼ ▼ ▼ ▼ ▼ ▼ ▼ ▼ ▼ ▼

BECAUSE YOU MAY FEEL more energetic on some days than on others, it is important to respect what your body wants to do, as opposed to what your brain wants you to do. This section gives some general pointers and then eight sequences with specific themes to help direct your practice.

Practice Guidelines

Here are answers to some common questions about practicing yoga.

Should I consult with my doctor or therapist? Before starting yoga, show this book to your doctor or therapist, and discuss your intentions for yoga practice to make sure they are appropriate for you. Check back at subsequent appointments to let your doctor or therapist know how your yoga is coming along.

How can I practice safely? It is not uncommon for those with fibromyalgia to have related or unrelated physical problems. Those that may affect your yoga practice include disk disease, sciatica, knee pain, and glaucoma. To make sure you practice safely, including during pregnancy, I have included a section called "Practice with Care" for each pose or exercise, where appropriate.

How often should I practice yoga? Whenever you begin a new exercise program, it is a good idea to commit to it for a number of days over a set period of time so you can notice any changes that are taking place. Practicing yoga only once a week may not result in many benefits except the moments of stretching or relaxation felt at that time.

Start out with at least two or three planned days per week. Decide what time of day is best for you; early mornings or evenings are good for many people. The duration and sequences of poses and movements can vary, depending on the needs of your body that day. It is very important to listen to your body and not to push it, yet you also want to receive the benefits. There may be days when Relaxation Pose (or Relaxation Pose with Chair or Side-Lying Relaxation Pose) is enough. Remember to start slowly with a short routine and build as you progress. Hopefully you will get to the point where you look forward to your practice because it makes you feel better!

Is a yoga class better than working on my own? Both are valuable. Working on your own gives you some quiet time and builds your self-confidence. Attending yoga classes with a qualified teacher can also be beneficial. The added bonus of practicing with other people, which can be fun, can sometimes be inspiring, too. Make sure your teacher has experience working with people who have special needs. Explain what your limitations are. If the type of yoga being taught is either too challenging or not to your liking, try a different style or class. Some more advanced yoga classes may also involve aerobic activity, so experiment and try different classes. If you feel peer pressure to keep up during a class, maybe that class isn't appropriate for you. Don't forget to listen to your body, and always check with your doctor or health care provider before starting any exercise class.

Where and when should I practice? When you are practicing on your own, it is helpful to have a room or corner in your home dedicated to yoga. If you're unable to designate a space, then store your props and bring them out for practice. If possible, practice in the same space and at the same time every day. To enhance your practice, let your housemates know that this is your practice time, turn off the phone, and dim the lights during Relaxation Pose.

Can I eat before practice? It is best to practice on an empty stomach, because you don't want to compress your abdomen while you are digesting food. Avoid eating a large meal for at least two hours beforehand.

What should I wear? Choose clothing that does not restrict your movements. These can be tights and leotards, or shorts or sweatpants with an elastic waist and a T-shirt. Your feet should be bare so you can feel the floor. Be comfortable. Take off your wristwatch. Remove your glasses during Relaxation Pose.

What if I have difficulty getting onto the floor? You have three options. (1) You can practice on your bed instead of the floor. (2) You can use the support of a sturdy piece of furniture, such as a desk, a sofa, or a bed, to help you get onto the floor. Place your mat near the support and put a folded blanket on the mat to cushion your knees. Center yourself in Mountain Pose before going further. Then place your dominant hand on the support and your other hand on the opposite thigh. Bend the knee on the supported side and place it on the blanket. Then lower your other knee. Place both hands in front of you on the floor, and sit onto one hip. Then lie on your stomach or roll onto your back. Reverse the process to come up. Do not try this if it hurts your knees or lower back. (3) Some poses offer a seated alternative to the floor version, such as Seated Cobra Pose.

What if I feel light-headed? If you feel light-headed when getting onto the floor, when lifting your head, or when moving from pose to pose, then go slowly or pause until it passes.

Do I really need props? Yes. A prop is a tool that supports your body, either to facilitate a stretch or to assist you when you are feeling tired. You can use items from around your house or props that have been designed for yoga (see Resources). Gather your props before you begin your practice, so you can focus on the poses and not tire yourself by looking for props between poses. The following props are used in this book:

- 1 nonskid mat (often called a yoga mat)
- 1 folding chair
- 1 adjustable yoga strap (or nonstretchy bathrobe belt)
- 1 small pillow (or towel)
- 2 firm blankets
- 1 bolster
- open wall space

Sequences

Now we are ready to put it all together. I have designed eight sequences that take up specific themes: four for pain relief, one to improve sleep and reduce fatigue, and three for maintaining general flexibility and body awareness. The timings for the poses are not specified, except for the three relaxation poses, which I encourage you to do for 5 to 10 minutes. In general, let how long you hold each pose be guided by your fatigue level or needs of the moment. Listen to your body. In each pose, visualize the area of the body you are working on. This can increase the effectiveness of your yoga. Focus on expanding the areas that are being stretched when you inhale, and soften and relax those areas when you exhale. Choose the sequence below that best fits your needs each day.

For General Pain Relief

These four gentle yoga poses may help relieve general body pain:

- Seated Mountain Pose, Figure 1
- Breathing Awareness, Figure 2A and Figure 2B
- Mountain Pose, Figure 3A and Figure 3B
- Relaxation Pose, Figure 24 (or Relaxation Pose with Chair, Figure 25, or Side-Lying Relaxation Pose, Figure 26)

Breathing affects your entire system and also can reflect stress in your body. For example, notice how your breath seems to be shorter and faster when you are in scary or stressful situations. Slowing your breathing and deepening each breath can help lower blood pressure and reduce stress. Stress often exacerbates pain. So an easy way to alleviate pain is to focus on your breathing, which can be done anywhere, anytime. Follow the guidelines for proper breathing techniques in part 2. As a variation, try to make the duration of each breath slower than the previous one. Count silently how long an inhalation takes, make the exhalation the same count, then make the next breath one count longer, and so on. Counting is also a way to keep your mind focused on something other than your pain. You can increase the number of breaths as long you feel comfortable.

Mountain Pose works on balance and posture. It can help you recognize where you feel discomfort or where you need to make adjustments. Often you can discover where you hold tension and release it in this pose. If standing is not an option or if you are not feeling up to practicing it standing, you can work in Seated Mountain Pose. Make sure your legs are relaxed and your pelvis is properly aligned, using your pelvis as your foundation instead of your feet.

According to the National Fibromyalgia Association, "Relaxation is an important tool to help the fibromyalgia patient deal with pain, sleep problems, and anxiety. Relaxation techniques can help calm the mind, slow the heart rate, and encourage deep, steady breathing." The guided instructions for the relaxation poses in part 2 and the Healing Breath that follows can be very helpful. Relaxing in a comfortable seated or prone position and listening to soothing music can also be beneficial. Many relaxation CDs are available online, in health food stores, and in bookstores. Having a variety of CDs can be valuable, as your moods and needs vary. Some guided visualizations focus on images other than the body; see what works best for you. The same relaxation may not suit you every day in every situation, so experiment. (See the Resources section for some suggestions.) Five minutes of relaxation can be enough for some people, but for many at least 10 minutes is advisable. Try to practice either Relaxation Pose or Relaxation Pose with Chair or Side-Lying Relaxation Pose once every day. See how much better you'll feel.

For Upper Body Pain Relief

Some fibromyalgia-related pain is directly associated with specific tense muscles. When stretching, keep your body warm, because cold promotes tensing. Move slowly, and breathe into the painful area. Remember to always work both sides of the body to keep balanced, even if the pain is only on one side.

It isn't necessary to practice all of these poses. If you do the seated variation, it is not necessary to do the standing one, and vice versa. Find the pose that matches the area where you are feeling pain.

NECK

* Neck Rotation Stretch, Figure 4
* Forward-and-Back Neck Stretch, Figure 5A and Figure 5B
* Ear-to-Shoulder Neck Stretch, Figure 6A and Figure 6B

TORSO

* Seated Mountain Pose, Figure 1
* Seated Eagle Pose, Figure 7A and Figure 7B
* Cobra Pose, Figure 10A and Figure 10B
* Seated Cobra Pose, Figure 11
* Cat Pose, Figure 12A and Figure 12B
* Reclining Twist Pose, Figure 17
* Seated Twist Pose, Figure 18A and Figure 18B

WRISTS

- Prayer Pose, Figure 8
- Reverse Prayer Pose, Figure 9

RELAXATION

- Legs-Up-the-Wall Pose, Figure 23
- Side-Lying Relaxation Pose, Figure 26
- Relaxation Pose with Chair, Figure 25
- Relaxation Pose, Figure 24

The three neck stretches each work on specific parts of the neck. Move very slowly and with awareness, making sure to breathe into each movement. Seated Mountain Pose helps release tension from your low back, while providing postural adjustments. A favorite pose for many of my students is Seated Eagle Pose, because it stretches the muscles around the shoulder blades in the upper back. Cobra Pose extends the back while opening the chest and can help your breathing. Cat Pose is a wonderful movement that opens the chest and stretches the shoulders and entire back. It teaches your body how to move the pelvis forward and back without any stress, to release the hips and lower back. Reclining Twist Pose and Seated Twist Pose rotate the spine and work especially on the lower back. It is also important to keep your wrists as flexible as possible. Stretching both the tops and undersides keeps the circulation open in your hands and should be incorporated into your daily routine. And, as my students well know, Relaxation Pose is one of the best ways to use your mind to change how it interprets pain. If you are too tired to practice poses, then at least treat yourself to some moments of relaxation.

For Lower Body Pain Relief

These poses and exercises can help ease specific lower body pain.

THIGHS

- Reclining Hamstring Stretch Pose, Figure 15A and Figure 15B
- Seated Hamstring Stretch Pose, Figure 16
- Reclining Thread-the-Needle, Figure 19A and Figure 19B
- Seated Thread-the-Needle, Figure 20
- Dancer Pose, Figure 21A, Figure 21B, and Figure 21C
- Side-Lying Dancer Pose, Figure 22

CALVES

- Downward-Facing Dog Pose, Figure 13
- Half Dog Pose, Figure 14A and Figure 14B and Figure 14C

RELAXATION

- Relaxation Pose with Chair, Figure 25
- Side-Lying Relaxation Pose, Figure 26

Remember to choose the appropriate poses or stretches and work slowly and gently. When you have tightness or pain in the backs of your thighs, Reclining Hamstring Stretch and Seated Hamstring Stretch can bring relief. Thread-the-Needle works on opening the hips and buttock muscles. Dancer Pose stretches the front thighs, and Downward-Facing Dog Pose and Half Dog Pose lengthen your calves. Relaxation Pose with Chair improves circulation to your legs, while also allowing your whole body to release. And of course I always recommend relaxation for pain relief.

Visualization for Pain Relief: The Healing Breath

There are many styles of visualization; you can find some good ones in the Resources section at the back of this book. If you use visualization while working in a pose or exercise, it can amplify the results. You can practice visualization most effectively in these poses:

* Seated Mountain Pose, Figure 1
* Relaxation Pose, Figure 24
* Relaxation Pose with Chair, Figure 25
* Side-Lying Relaxation Pose, Figure 26

A guided visualization that I have found to be effective in reducing general or specific pain is what I call the Healing Breath. Read the instructions that follow until you can remember them before beginning. Or you might want to have someone read this section to you or tape yourself reading it, so you can listen while relaxing.

Begin in one of the poses listed and make sure you are comfortable. Inhale and exhale slowly, focusing on how the air feels as it passes through your nose, into your body, and back out. Think of your breath as the gift of life—prana: life force. Let it feel soothing as it flows inside. If you have general pain, visualize this healing breath filling your whole body. If your pain is more specific, on the inhalations, bring the breath directly to your pain. Then, for either type of pain, let each new inhalation bring energy to expand and soften, cleanse and release, rejuvenate. With the exhalations, let the tensions and heaviness of your pain flow out with the breath. Breathe slowly, and continue until you feel quiet, heavy, and more relaxed. Come out of the pose when you are ready. Notice the difference you have made in yourself.

For Reducing Fatigue and Improving Sleep

Disturbed, nonrestorative sleep can cause fatigue. (See part 4 on the importance of sleep, for further information.) Before going to bed, do some gentle stretches in the areas that seem especially tense (as described above). But relaxation techniques are the most important practice to do before sleep:

- Relaxation Pose with Chair, Figure 25
- Relaxation Pose, Figure 24
- Side-Lying Relaxation Pose, Figure 26

If you choose Relaxation Pose with Chair, you release any lower back tension while letting yourself slow down. But from that position you will then need to get up to go to bed. You might prefer practicing Relaxation Pose in bed with pillows under your knees, which is a good position to release tension and encourage a deeper sleep. Then you don't have to move and can just drift off to sleep. Some of my students use music to enhance their relaxation. Keep the player by the bed, and set it to shut off automatically, so sleep can follow without distraction. See what works best for you.

SEATED BEGINNER SEQUENCE

If you are not experiencing pain or discomfort but want to practice from a chair, here is a beginning routine done seated, except for Relaxation Pose with Chair.

- Seated Mountain Pose, Figure 1
- Breathing Awareness, Figure 2
- Neck Rotation Stretch, Figure 4
- Forward-and-Back Neck Stretch, Figure 5A and Figure 5B
- Ear-to-Shoulder Neck Stretch, Figure 6
- Prayer Pose, Figure 8
- Reverse Prayer Pose, Figure 9
- Seated Cobra Pose, Figure 11
- Seated Hamstring Stretch Pose, Figure 16
- Seated Twist Pose, Figure 18A and Figure 18B
- Relaxation Pose with Chair, Figure 25

BEGINNER MAINTENANCE SEQUENCE

If you are not experiencing pain or discomfort but want a routine shorter than the complete sequence, you can practice this routine.

- Breathing Awareness, Figure 2
- Mountain Pose, Figure 3
- Neck Rotation Stretch, Figure 4
- Forward-and-Back Neck Stretch, Figure 5A and Figure 5B
- Ear-to-Shoulder Neck Stretch, Figure 6
- Prayer Pose, Figure 8
- Reverse Prayer Pose, Figure 9
- Cat Pose, Figure 12A and Figure 12B
- Seated Hamstring Stretch, Figure 16
- Seated Twist Pose, Figure 18A and Figure 18B
- Relaxation Pose, Figure 24

Full Maintenance Sequence

If you are not experiencing pain or discomfort, you can follow the complete sequence of poses in part 2 to maintain flexibility and body awareness. You can decide whether to practice both the standing and seated variations of those poses that offer both. You can always start slowly and build up over time.

Practicing the Beginner Maintenance Sequence or the Full Maintenance Sequence, if you are up to it, at least three times a week is optimal. If this seems too rigorous, do what you can, until you build up the strength to practice the complete series. On days when you do not have the time or energy, practice the sequence for General Pain Relief. These stress-reducers have the most generalized effect, using the least physical effort. Ideally, besides the three days of your sequence routine, try to practice at least 10 to 20 minutes on the other days. Choose whatever poses your body seems to want to do. And if you don't have 10 minutes, then do 5. Deciding that every day you will do something good for your body is a big step. Don't make more demands than you can realistically handle. Look forward to your practice, knowing you are taking charge and learning to help yourself feel better!

Part IV:

Living with Fibromyalgia

▼　▼　▼　▼　▼　▼　▼　▼　▼　▼

THE SYMPTOMS OF FIBROMYALGIA vary from person to person and often from day to day. Fatigue and general body pain can be pervasive. These lifestyle suggestions may help you live more comfortably, with reduced symptoms.

The Importance of Sleep

Imagine sleeping for only a few hours one night, and maybe the next night getting no sleep, then a few hours again the next night. You would feel totally exhausted! This is how many people with fibromyalgia feel all the time, because they don't get the deep, restorative sleep we all need. Disturbed sleep is common in 86 to 90 percent of people diagnosed with fibromyalgia, according to a publication of the National Fibromyalgia Association. The result, of course, is sleepiness during the day and less energy for ordinary activities. So whatever you can do to improve your sleep is vitally important.

Following some general rules can help your sleep. Go to bed at a regular time every night to help support your body's natural rhythms. Your bed and bedroom should be as comfortable as possible. Make sure your pillow or style of bed is not provoking any discomfort. Keep the room temperature moderate, so you are neither too hot nor too cold. Do not drink liquids too close to bedtime, so you won't have to go to the bathroom in the night. Try not to do any activities before bed that increase anxiety or alertness. Avoid going to bed with a full stomach. Do some gentle stretching to relieve muscle tension (see part 3). For some people, a warm bath and soft music can help reduce stress before bed. Using relaxation techniques can be very beneficial (see part 3). Some common and prescription drugs, including beta-blockers, stimulating antidepressants, corticosteroids, and decongestants, such as some cold and allergy medications, can disrupt sleep. You should talk with your doctor to see if any sleep medications are advisable.

Nutrition

Good nutrition is important for maintaining general health, but it can be confusing to know what diet to follow and whether to take supplements. Talk with your doctor or health care practitioner to find out what is best for you.

Since fatigue and poor sleep are common fibromyalgia symptoms, learn about the foods that affect these conditions. Caffeine, for example, should be avoided, especially in the late afternoon or evening. It increases the level of adrenaline in the blood, which causes an increase in heart rate, breathing rate, urinary output, and the production of stomach acids. All of these are the opposite of what you want when you're trying to go to sleep.

Going to bed with a full stomach is also not advisable, as it requires your system to go to work to digest just as you're trying to slow down and sleep.

So avoid heavy meals late in the day. Also, since foods that are high in fat are harder to digest, they should be eaten early and avoided at night. Choose foods that help you relax. Again, talk with your health care practitioner, and experiment to learn what works best for you.

Exercise

Exercise is essential for decreasing fibromyalgia symptoms. People who gently exercise two to five times a week experience a 25 percent reduction in symptoms. Aerobic exercise keeps the heart strong, so try to add some gentle aerobics to your day. Aerobics is any activity that increases your heart rate. But not all aerobic exercises are appropriate for persons with fibromyalgia. High-impact aerobics can stress your joints and cause more muscle pain, so choose low-impact exercises, such as brisk walking, biking, swimming, water aerobics, and low-impact aerobics classes. Classes that are aimed at the older population contain less jumping, so programs like People with Arthritis Can Exercise (PACE), offered through the Arthritis Foundation, might be good ones to check out.

It is important to start your exercise program slowly. At first, exercise may make your pain worse. While some muscle soreness is normal when you start to exercise, sharp pain may be a sign that you have overworked your muscles. As you progress, exercise will become more comfortable. For exercise to help, you have to do it regularly. Start small and keep going. Eventually you'll get relief from pain and start sleeping better.

Well-known rheumatologist Daniel Clauw advises focusing on low-impact exercises and beginning with only five minutes, three or four times a week, increasing by a minute or two each week. If you are intolerant of exercise because it worsens symptoms, warm-water aquatic therapy can be a good way of starting a movement program. Dr. Clauw says he eventually likes to get patients up to twenty minutes of aerobic exercise every day, and he tells them it will typically take three to four months to reach this point. So don't be overly ambitious or push too hard at the beginning, because you may get discouraged if you don't feel good right away or if you get too tired. Remember to build up slowly and listen to your body.

Movement in Daily Life

Often when you are coping with the symptoms of fibromyalgia, exercise is not at all appealing. However, as is true for almost everyone, moving to our capacity keeps us lively and can improve our quality of life. The old saying "use it or lose it" does hold some truth. Try to make your daily life less sedentary. Work in your garden, dance, walk your dog, take the long way around the mall. Here are some tips for aiding daily movement:

- Prioritize your chores and do them for shorter time periods, so you won't get too fatigued.
- Minimize repetitive movements and overhead work.
- Use short strokes when vacuuming or sweeping.
- Take smaller steps when walking downhill.
- Use the stairs to add exercise to your day (unless you have hip, knee, or ankle limitations).
- Pay attention to your posture and your breath.
- Stretch and relax daily.
- Pay attention to signals from your body.

Another option that can be helpful is to consult an occupational therapist. They are trained to help you find ways to continue with the daily activities of life, such as dressing, cleaning, and shopping. The key is to get up off the couch and keep moving.

Psychological Well-Being

Learning to live with your symptoms is often not easy, but your mental state can greatly influence how you feel. It can have a big effect on your physical pain, making it more or less bearable. Modern medicine does not have the magic pill to make your fibromyalgia disappear, but you can use your mind to help you cope more positively. Stress and anger add tension to the body, which can increase symptoms. So anger management, stress reduction, and getting help with depression can improve your ability to live better with fibromyalgia.

Be good to yourself, and do something every day that you love. Listen to your favorite music, buy yourself fresh flowers, write in a daily journal, relax, do what makes you happy. Smile. Feeling happy is good for your health.

Living well with fibromyalgia means finding the right amount of sleep, exercise, nutrition, and psychological or spiritual fulfillment. Find health care practitioners who understand how to support all of these. Then it is up to you. Only you can make time to play, rest, and enjoy your life.

Yoga with Shoosh Lettick Crotzer

Shoosh Lettick Crotzer offers ongoing yoga classes in Morro Bay and San Luis Obispo, California. She also teaches workshops and gives presentations on yoga for persons with special needs, such as arthritis, multiple sclerosis, and cancer. For more information, email her at shsh@mobilityltd.com.

DVDs and CD

By Shoosh Lettick Crotzer, produced and distributed by her company, Mobility Limited, (800) 366–6038, www.mobilityltd.com.

Yoga for Arthritis: Pathways to Better Living with Arthritis & Related Conditions (DVD)

Yoga for MS and Related Conditions: Pathways Exercise Video for People with Limited Mobility (DVD)

Rest Easy: Three Guided Relaxation Routines to Help Reduce Stress (CD)

Props and Clothing Photographed in Yoga for Fibromyalgia

Props: Hugger-Mugger Yoga Products, (800) 473-4888, www.huggermugger.com

Clothing: Marie Wright Yoga Wear, (800) 217-0006, www.mariewright.com

Chair: Meco Corporation, (800) 251-7558, www.meco.net

Other Recommended Resources

BOOKS

Fransen, Jenny, R.N., and I. John Russell, M.D., Ph.D. *The Fibromyalgia Help Book: Practical Guide to Living Better with Fibromyalgia*. St. Paul, MN: Smith House Press, 1996.

Iyengar, B.K.S. *Light on Yoga*. New York: Schocken Books, 1995.

Lasater, Judith, Ph.D., P.T. *Relax and Renew: Restful Yoga for Stressful Times*. Berkeley, CA: Rodmell Press, 1995. (800) 841-3123, www.rodmellpress.com.

Mehta, Silva, Mira Mehta, and Shyam Mehta. *Yoga: The Iyengar Way*. New York: Knopf, 1990.

Pellegrino, Mark J., M.D. *Fibromyalgia: Up Close and Personal*. Columbus, OH: Anadem Publisher, Inc, 2005.

Schatz, Mary Pullig, M.D. *Back Care Basics*, Berkeley, CA: Rodmell Press, 1992. (800) 841-3123, www.rodmellpress.com.

Schiffmann, Erich. *Yoga: The Spirit and Practice of Moving into Stillness*. New York: Pocket Books, 1996.

Williamson, Miryam Ehrlich. *Fibromyalgia: A Comprehensive Approach*. New York: Walker and Co., 1996.

White, Ganga. *Yoga Beyond Belief: Insights to Awaken and Deepen Your Practice*. Berkeley, CA: North Atlantic Books, 2007.

MAGAZINES

Arthritis Practitioner
www.arthritispractitioner.com

Fibromyalgia AWARE
www.fmaware.org/magazine.html

Yoga + Joyful Living
www.himalayaninstitute.org/yogaplus

Yoga Journal
www.yogajournal.com

RELAXATION CDs

Halpern, Steven. *Music for Healing: Body, Mind and Spirit*
    www.therelaxationcompany.com

Miller, Emmett, M.D., with Halpern, Steven, *Letting Go of Stress*
    www.drmiller.com

Folan, Lilias. *Lilias! Discover Serenity: A Guided Relaxation Program*
    www.liliasyoga.com

White, Ganga, and Rich, Tracey. *Meditation Is Your Life*
    www.whitelotus.org

WHERE TO FIND A YOGA TEACHER

www.yogaalliance.com

www.yogajournal.com

www.yogateacherassoc.org

It is important to discuss your limitations and goals with your doctor and then
with your yoga teacher before beginning any class. Most public yoga classes are
not geared specifically toward therapeutic yoga. I recommend that you find a
qualified teacher to work with one-on-one at first or look for workshops that
address your specific limitations and needs.

About the Author

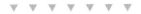

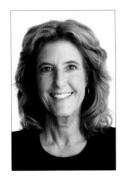SHOOSH LETTICK CROTZER has been teaching yoga since 1974 and now specializes in working with students with special needs. She has a masters degree in diagnostic education. In 1994, while teaching for the National MS Society, she founded the production and distribution company Mobility Limited and wrote and produced the video *Yoga for MS*. She wrote and produced *Yoga for Arthritis* in partnership with the Arthritis Foundation in 1997. She has given workshops and made presentations on yoga and arthritis at international rheumatology conferences.

Shoosh began her yoga training in India in the 1970s and continued with Sivananda Yoga teachers in Los Angeles. She has a background in Iyengar-style yoga and has studied with Joel Kramer, Ganga White, and Tracey Rich.

Shoosh has taught yoga at universities, yoga centers, health clubs, and privately throughout the country. She is the founder and director of the nonprofit organization Enhancement, Inc., which works to improve the quality of life for breast cancer survivors. She lives in Morro Bay, California, with her husband, Colby.

DEIRDRE CARRIGAN has been teaching yoga since 1987 in San Francisco Bay Area health clubs, yoga and fitness studios, workplaces, and private homes. Her primary teacher is Donald Moyer. She graduated from the Advanced Studies Program at The Yoga Room, in Berkeley, California, and joined the faculty there. In addition to her ongoing classes, Deirdre has led yoga workshops in San Francisco and at Tassajara Zen Mountain Center. She currently resides at Green Gulch Farm, studying Zen meditation.

Deirdre first experienced symptoms of fibromyalgia in 1989. It took many years for her to receive a diagnosis and medical treatment, during which time her practice of yoga helped her recover her balance and energy. She credits yoga with allowing her to maintain an extensive teaching schedule.

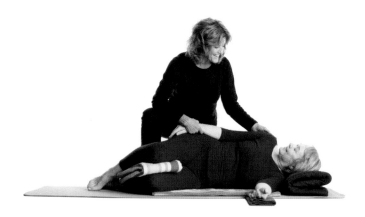

From the Publisher

▼ ▼ ▼ ▼ ▼ ▼ ▼

RODMELL PRESS PUBLISHES books on yoga, Buddhism, aikido, and Taoism. In the Bhagavadgita it is written, "Yoga is skill in action." It is our hope that our books will help individuals develop a more skillful practice—one that brings peace to their daily lives and to the earth.

We thank those whose support, encouragement, and practical advice sustain us in our efforts. In particular, we are grateful to Reb Anderson, B. K. S. Iyengar, Wendy Palmer, and Yvonne Rand for their inspiration.

Catalog Request

(510) 841-3123 or (800) 841-3123

(510) 841-3123 (fax)

info@rodmellpress.com

www.rodmellpress.com

Trade Sales/United States, International

Publishers Group West

(800) 788-3123 • (510) 528-5511 (sales fax)

info@pgw.com • www.pgw.com

Foreign Language and Book Club Rights

Linda Cogozzo, Publisher

(510) 841-3123

linda@rodmellpress.com

www.rodmellpress.com

Index

▼ ▼ ▼ ▼ ▼ ▼ ▼